Materials in Restorative Dentistry

Edited by

A. Parameswaran
K.S. Karthikeyan

CBS

CBS PUBLISHERS & DISTRIBUTORS
4596/1-A, 11 Darya Ganj, New Delhi - 110 002 (India)

ISBN : 81-239-0706-0

First Edition : 1998
First Reprint : 2000
Second Reprint : 2001

Published by :
Satish Kumar Jain for CBS Publishers & Distributors,
4596/1A, 11 Darya Ganj, New Delhi - 110 002 (India)

Printed at :
Asia Printograph, Shahdara,
Delhi - 110 032 (India)

TABLE OF CONTENTS

CONTRIBUTORS

1. **Dr. ANNAPOORNI, H.**
Professor
Department of Prosthodontics,
Meenakshi Ammal Dental College, Chennai.

2. **Dr. BALAGOPAL, S.**
Professor
Department of Conservative Dentistry and Endodontics,
Saveetha Dental College, Chennai.

3. **Dr. JAGANNATHAN, K.**
Reader
Department of Conservative Dentistry and Endodontics,
Ragas Dental College, Chennai.

4. **Dr. KANDASWAMY, D.**
Reader
Department of Conservative Dentistry and Endodontics,
Tamil Nadu Government Dental College, Chennai.

5. **Dr. KARTHIKEYAN, K.S.**
Professor
Department of Conservative Dentistry and Endodontics,
Meenakshi Ammal Dental College, Chennai.

6. **Dr. LAKSHMI NARAYANAN, L.**
Professor and Head of Department,
Department of Conservative Dentistry and Endodontics,
Saveetha Dental College, Chennai.

7. **Dr. PARAMESWARAN, A.**
Professor and Head of Department,
Department of Conservative Dentistry and Endodontics,
Meenakshi Ammal Dental College, Chennai.

8. **Dr. SOLOMON, E.G.R.**
Post Graduate Professor of Prosthodontics,
A.B. Shetty Memorial Institute of Dental Sciences,
Mangalore.

9. **Dr. SUBBA RAO, C.V.**
Professor and Head of Department,
Department of Conservative Dentistry and Endodontics,
Tamil Nadu Government Dental College, Chennai.

10. **Dr. SUKUMARAN, V.G.**
Professor and Head of Department,
Department of Conservative Dentistry and Endodontics,
Balaji Dental College, Chennai.

11. **Dr. SURESH CHANDRA, B.**
Vice-Principal, Professor and Head of Department,
Department of Conservative Dentistry and Endodontics,
A.B. Shetty Memorial Institute of Dental Sciences,
Mangalore.

12. **Dr. SUSILA, V.**
Lecturer,
Department of Conservative Dentistry and Endodontics,
Meenakshi Ammal Dental College, Chennai.

INTRODUCTION

Materials used in dentistry are being developed, giving more importance to lasting service and esthetics. The text material of this monograph is focussing on a variety of aspects of dental materials and its acceptance by the human tissues as a whole. All these chapters are detailed and presented by renouned teachers of Conservative Dentistry and Prosthodontics to convey the current information from research and clinical experience.

This monograph consists of articles presented on 27thand 28th Feb'98 at the "***Postgraduate meet – '98"*** at Meenakshi Ammal Dental College, Chennai. These articles enumerate contemporary restorative materials and its application in various restorative procedures. The points of importance in handling modern materials are stressed in detail, such as Polyalkeonate cements which are trying to capture the prime place in restorative practice. Many finer aspects of luting Cements are enumerated with graphic illustrations. The time tested materials like Ceramics, Gold and Amalgam are also presented to review its extensive usage in restorative dentisıry. *"A Compendium on Titanium – The wonder metal"* is included. Application of materiais as substitutes within human tissues are to be done with caution, particularly when used as a Root end filling material. Acceptance and tolerance of these dental materials are discussed.

We express our gratitute to **Mr. A.N. RADHAKRISHNAN** of Meenakshi Ammal Trust for his liberal financial support and co-operation in bringing out this monograph. The principal of the institution, **Dr. E. MUNIRATHNAM NAIDU** has taken active part in initiating this primary academic activity, for the benifit of the post graduate students of Conservative Dentistry & Endodontics and Prosthodontics.

We take this opportunity to thank the Vice - Chancellor of Tamil Nadu Dr. M.G.R. Medical University, **Dr.(MAJOR) D.RAJA** MS(ortho)., D.Ortho, FIAS, FMSA, who has inagurated the ***"Post***

Graduate Meet – '98" and the former Vice Chancellor of Tamil Nadu Dr. M.G.R Medical University **Dr. B.P. RAJAN** B.Sc, MDS, FICD who has released the monograph on this occasion.

Our thanks are due to the members of faculty for their valuble contributions. The post–graduate students, **Dr. Aby Mammen** and **Dr. K. Senthil Kumar** for their help in proof reading and **Mr. Mahesh Kumar,** for the printing and the presentation of this monograph.

Feb 27th 1998

A.P.
K.S.K.

METAL CERAMIC SYSTEM - MATERIAL AND TECHNICAL CONSIDERATIONS

Annapoorni H.

The ceramic anterior restoration though highly aesthetic, are brittle and subject to fracture from high tensile stresses or impact, and an all metal restoration is only an acceptable posterior restoration.

A wise combination of these is the metal ceramic restoration, which consists of a strong metal substrate or coping on to which aesthetic ceramic is fused. This was developed as early as 1950 and since its introduction it has been called by varying names, as Ceramco crown, Porcelain veneer crown (PVC), Porcelain fused to gold (PFG), Porcelain fused to metal (PFM). Metal ceramic is a more precise term.

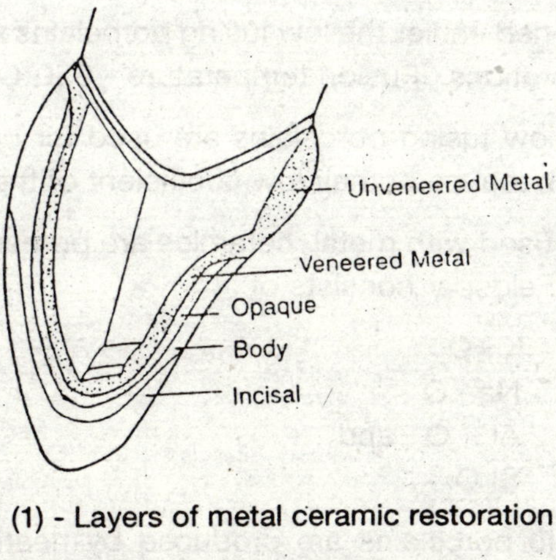

Fig (1) - Layers of metal ceramic restoration

The development of ceramic metal restoration was made possible because of the following :

1. Low fusing ceramics.
2. High fusing alloys.
3. Ceramics and alloys that have matching coefficients of thermal expansion.

4. Ceramics and alloys that form a strong bond.

MATERIAL SCIENCE

The most important criteria in the selection of ceramics for cast metal restoration is that the ceramic must fuse to the alloy without warping of the metal, and on cooling of ceramic and metal they must contract in unision, so that the ceramic does not crack.

Porcelain is a composite of crystalline minerals such as silica, feldspar and alumina in an amorphous matrix of glass.

Opaque oxides such as titanium oxide, zirconium oxide and tin oxide are added to the translucent glass to diffuse light transmission and simulate the appearance of natural teeth.

According to their fusion range, porcelain is divided into :
High Fusing
Medium Fusing
Low Fusing
Ultra Low Fusing

As mentioned earlier the low fusing porcelains are used in metal ceramic restorations. (Fusion temperature - 950°C-1020°C)

The ultra low fusing porcelains are used for crown and bridge with titanium because of their low coefficient of thermal expansion.

Porcelain used with metal ceramics are primarily "Feldspathic Porcelains". Feldspar consists of :

Potash	K_2O
Soda	Na_2O
Alumina	Al_2O_3 and
Silica	SiO_2

Feldspathic porcelains are produced by heating a mixture of sodium feldspar and potassium feldspar at very high temperature and then immediately quenching it.

This process is repeated several times, resulting in the formation of a glassy phase composed of $Si\text{-}O_2$ network and a crystalline phase composed of leucite ($K_2O.\ Al_2O_3.\ 4SiO_2$). Hence these porcelains are also called **Leucite Porcelains.** Leucite has a very high co-efficient of thermal expansion. It should be noted that feldspar is not present in the final product nor is it necessary as raw material to produce leucite crystals.

GLASS MODIFIERS

Glass modifiers can be defined as elements that interfere with $Si\text{-}O_2$ (glass) network and alter their three dimensional state. This reduces the coefficient of thermal expansion of porcelains.

Alkali metal ions such as sodium, potassium and calcium may be added as glass modifiers. Higher concentration of glass modifiers have disastrous results such as reduced resistance of glass to attack by water, acids and alkalis. Further more devitrification of glass may take place during firing (i.e) the glassy network crystalises.

Other additions to these porcelains are metallic oxides which are added to obtain various shades of porcelains. These are also called stain, surface colorants or characterisation porcelains. These oxides also act as glass modifiers.

The metal coping in a metal ceramic restoration is covered with three layers of porcelain (fig. 1)

1. Opaque Porcelain - This conceals the matter underneath and initiates the development of shade. It plays an important role in the development of bond between the porcelain and the matter. It consists of high concentrations of insoluble oxides such as titanium oxide and zirconium oxide.

2. Body Porcelain or Dentin Porcelain - This makes up for the bulk of the restoration providing most of the colour and shade. This is fired onto the opaque layer in conjunction with incisal porcelain.

3. Enamel or Incisal Porcelain - This imparts translucency to the restoration since it is translucent by itself and is influenced by the colour of the underlying body porcelain.

METAL CERAMIC ALLOYS

The alloys used in metal ceramics are classified broadly as

High Noble Alloys

Noble Alloys

Base Metal Alloys

THE HIGH NOBLE ALLOYS are those that contain at least 60% by weight of Noble Metals. These alloys are divided based on their composition into :

1. Gold Platinum Palladium Alloy
2. Gold palladium Silver Alloy
3. Gold Palladium Alloy

Gold Platinum Palladium Alloy

They consists of :

Gold	85-90%
Platinum	5-10%
Palladium	5-7%
Iron	0-1%
Indium	0-1%
Tin	0-1%

Gold promotes the handling characteristics of the alloy, while platinum hardens the gold. Palladium lowers the co-efficient of thermal expansion. Iron reacts with platinum to form a precipitate of FePt, while along with tin and indium help to create a bonding mechanism between porcelain and metal. These alloys are susceptible to sag deformation, therefore they must be preferably used in short span bridges, anterior cantilevers or crowns.

Gold Palladium Silver Alloy

These alloys may be again divided into two types based on their silver content. One that contains 12% weight of silver and the other that contains more than 12% by weight. They have the following composition :

Gold	50%
Silver	12%

Palladium	30%
Indium/tin	8%

Compared to the gold platinum system, these are more economical, harder and stronger.

Gold Palladium Alloy

These alloys are very expensive. The lack of silver decreases the co-efficient of thermal contraction. Therefore porcelains with low co-efficient of thermal contraction must be used. The advantage of this system is that greening of porcelain does not occur.

THE NOBLE ALLOYS are those that contain atleast 25% by weight of noble metals, but not necessarily contain any gold. Predominantly the noble alloys are the palladium based alloys. "These alloys are an excellent compromise between the High Noble Gold Alloy and the Base Metal Alloys". These alloys are moderately priced, workability is similar to that of gold and they have scrap value. Based on the composition they are divided into :

1. Palladium Silver Alloy
2. High Palladium Alloy
3. Palladium Copper Alloy
4. Palladium Cobalt Alloy
5. Palladium Gallium Alloy

Palladium Silver Alloy

The Pd-Ag alloy contains 50-60% of Pd and 20-40% of silver. Tin, Indium or both are added to increase hardness. In some of these alloys, formation of internal oxide rather than external oxide has been reported. This causes mechanical retention of porcelain rather than chemical retention. But this does not produce any significant clinical failure.

Because of higher amount of silver content, co-efficient of thermal contraction is lowered greening of procelain occurs.

'd-Ag-Sn System fig. (2) Internal Oxide formation

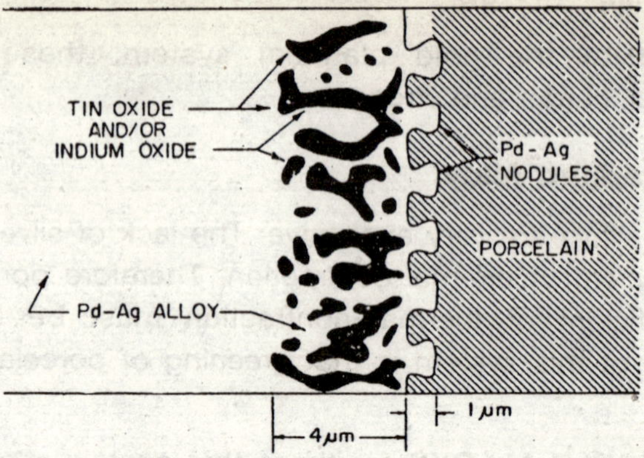

fig. (2) Pd-Ag-Sn System, Internal Oxide formation

High Palladium Alloy (75-90% of Pd)

These do not contain any silver and therefore greening of porcelain does not occur. Further more since Pd is costlier than silver, these alloys are more expensive.These alloys form a dark layer of surface oxide which is difficult to mask with opaque porcelain.

Palladium Copper Alloy

These alloys have the hardness of base metal alloys and are far easier to handle. Dark oxides are formed on the metal surface that may affect aesthetics unless wisely concealed by opaque porcelain. Studies are being conducted on the cytotoxic effect of copper released intraorally from Pd-Cu alloy.

Palladium Cobalt Alloy

This alloy is the most sag resistant among the noble metal alloys. It contains about 78-88% of palladium and 4-10% of cobalt. Some of the alloys contain gallium upto 8%. These alloys have very good handling characteristics. Discolouration of porcelain does occur, but is not of clinical significance.

Palladium Gallium Alloy

These alloys are of two types, one with silver and the other with silver & gold. They are the most recent of noble metals. The surface oxides produced by this group of metals is very light in colour.

The silver content is low and does not cause porcelain greening. The metal-ceramic bond with these alloys is being studied.

THE BASE METAL ALLOYS used in metal ceramic restoration are nickel based, cobalt based, pure titanium and titanium alloys.

Nickel Chromium Alloy

The Nickel-Chromium Alloy contains :

61 - 81 % by weight of Ni

10 - 28 % by weight of Cr

2 - 5 % by weight of Mb

Berrilium up to 1.8 % is added by some manufacturers. The Ni-Cr-Be alloy has retained its popularity in spite of the potential toxicity of Be, and allergic potential of Ni. Addition of Cr is essential to provide passivation and corrossion resistance. This addition increases the fusion temperature. Therefore addition of Be is prefered to decrease the fusion temperature of the alloy.

Cobalt Chromium Alloy

The Co-Cr Alloy used in metal ceramics contain

Cobalt	53-67%
Chromium	25-32%
Molybdenum	2- 6%

Some of these alloys also contain 3-6% of ruthenium, which is a noble metal. Ruthenium increases the castability. The principal difference between the cobalt based alloys formulated for partial denture work and metal ceramics is that, carbon is added for the former. This strengthens the alloy by carbide formation.Crown and bridge alloys are strengthened by solid solution hardening mechanisms.

Commercially Pure Titanium

Titanium is a light Silver-Grey metal with a S.G of 4.5 Gm/ cu.cm. Pure titanium is soft,weak and extremely ductile. Commercially pure titanium (CpTi) is an alpha alloy of titanium containing minor amounts of oxygen and nitrogen. This alloy is highly resistant to corrossion.

Titanium Alloy

The most commonly used titanium alloy for dental application is Ti-6Al-4V but CpTi are more popular as metal ceramic alloy. Both titanium and its alloys are gaining acceptance for dental use since they exhibit, bio-compatibility, corrosion resistance, low specific gravity, good mechanical property and low cost. However, titanium suffers from its violent reactivity with oxygen at high temperature that yields an excessively thick layer of TiO. This presents difficulty in porcelain bonding. Surface Nitridation of CpTi has proven to be effective in controlling the surface oxide thickness, thus ensuring satisfactory bonding with porcelain. CpTi and titanium alloy require specially formulated investments to minimise the interaction of molten metal with the investment.

Properties of Base Metal Alloys Versus Noble Metal Alloys

There is no doubt about the fact that the Noble metal alloys have far superior handling characteristics than the Base metal alloys.

The Base metal alloys have greater modulus of elasticity and hence greater rigidity. Therefore these alloys can be handled with greater ease in long span bridges where flexure may cause failure.Further more, high modulus of elasticity permits fabrication of thinner castings and so coping thickness can be reduced from 0.3mm recommended for noble metal alloys to a uniform thickness of 0.1mm in base metal alloy.

Biological problems have never been associated with gold alloys or palladium based alloys. However, nickel is one of the most common cause of allergic dermatitis and is believed to be responsible for more allergic reactions than all the other metals combined, and scrap cannot be reused. Inspite of its disadvantages, base metal alloys reign supreme as alloys of choice for metal ceramic restorations.

BONDING MECHANISMS

The primary requirement for the success of metal ceramic restoration is a strong bond between metal and porcelain.The mechanism of bonding porcelain to metal substructure is based on :

1. Vanderwaal's forces.
2. Chemical bonding.
3. Mechanical ineterlocking.
4. Compressive forces.

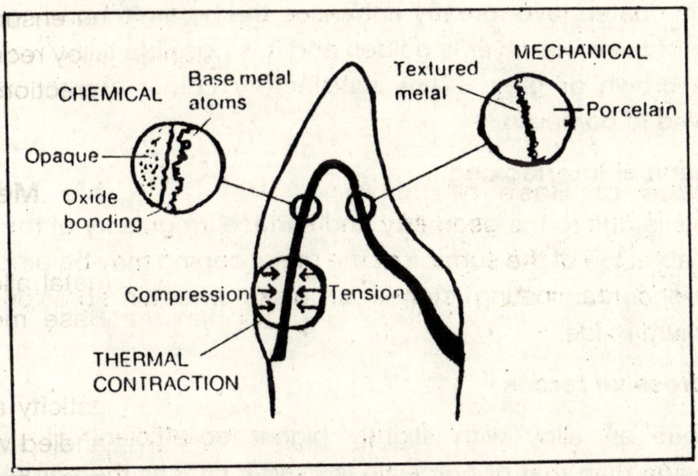

fig. (3) Bonding Mechanism

BONDING OF PORCELAIN TO METAL

Vanderwaals forces

It is based on mutual attraction of charged molecules. They do contribute to bonding but are not very significant. But it is very significant in the initiation of the most important mechanism, the chemical bond.

Chemical Bonding

Chemical bonding is primarily due to oxide layer formed on the external surface of the metal. It is essential to have an optimum thickness of oxide layer for effective bonding. In the case of gold alloys trace elements such as tin, indium or iron migrate to the surface of the metal during firing. They form oxides and bond with similar oxides present in porcelain. Base metal alloys readily form chromium oxides that bond to porcelain. Electrodeposition of metal coatings on the surface of copings and then heating to form metal oxides is one of the methods adopted to enhance bonding between porcelain and metal. One method is the deposition of a layer of pure gold on the coping followed by flash deposition of tin. This tin coated layer greatly enhances the ceramic bonding. The colour of the oxide layer is golden and it is possible to activate it to redish brown or grey. Thus satisfactory colour control can be achieved in porcelain.

Mechanical Interlocking

This is due to the geometry and surface irregularity of the alloy. Micro abrasion of the surface of the metal coping may be produced with noncontaminating stones or disks and air abrasion with aluminium oxide.

Compressive forces

When an alloy with slightly higher co-efficient of thermal expansion than that of porcelain is used it causes the porcelain to draw towards the coping when the restoration cools after firing. This contributes to the interfacial bond strength due to compressive stresses.

The most important requirement in forming a good interfacial bond is adequate wetting of the alloy surface by porcelain. Good wetting is associated with low contact angle. The contact between a dental porcelain and high noble alloy is reported to be 40-59 and for nickel base alloy it is 80-100%. These values are affected by furnace atmosphere.

TECHNICAL CONSIDERATIONS - Metal Ceramic Restoration

The Anterior Metal Ceramic Restoration

Indications:-

Extensive tooth destruction as a result of Caries.

Endodontically treated tooth.

Retainers for FPD.

Retainers for RPD.

Patients with reduced interaocclusal clearance or a strong masculatory masculature.

Peg shape laterals.

Whenever there is need for a greater retention and strength.

Contraindications:-

Whenever a more conservative restoration is possible, a metal ceramic restoration should not be thought of. In young patients with large pulp chamber the metal ceramic crown is contraindicated. Patients with active caries and untreated periodontal disease are not a good choice for MCR.

ARMAMENTARIUM

High speed hand piece
Flat end tapered diamond
Small wheel shaped diamond
Chamfer diamond (Torpedo diamond)
Chamfer bur (Torpedo bur)
No. 170 bur
Long thin tapered diamond

The porcelain fused metal restoration is a combination of metal and porcelain. Hence the preparation is also a combination. The first step is the placement of depth orientation grooves on the labial surface with the flat end tapering diamond. The labial grooves are cut in two sets. One set parallel to the gingival half and other set parallel to the incisal half of the labial surface. These groove should be 1.2 mm deep and incisally they should cut through and through, 2mm gingivally. See fig. (4)

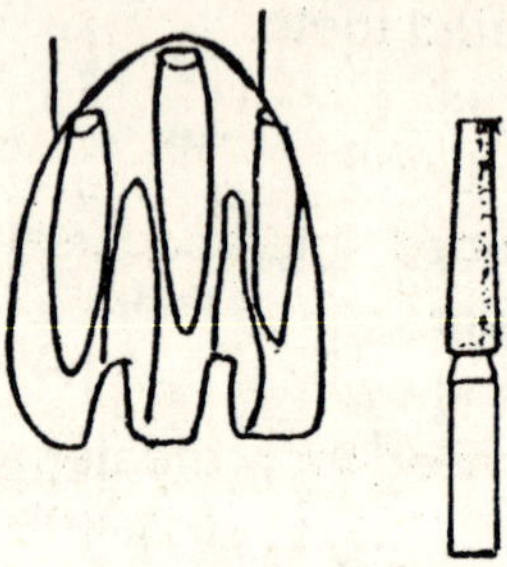

Fig (4)-Depth Orientation Grooves: *Flat end tapered diamond*

Incisal reduction : It is done with the same instrument such that it parallels the inclination of the unprepared incisal edge. It is mandatory to achieve incisal reduction as the first step so that good instrument access is obtained both to the axial surface and the gingival finish line. Adequate incisal reduction is necessary to obtain good incisal translucency of the finished restoration.

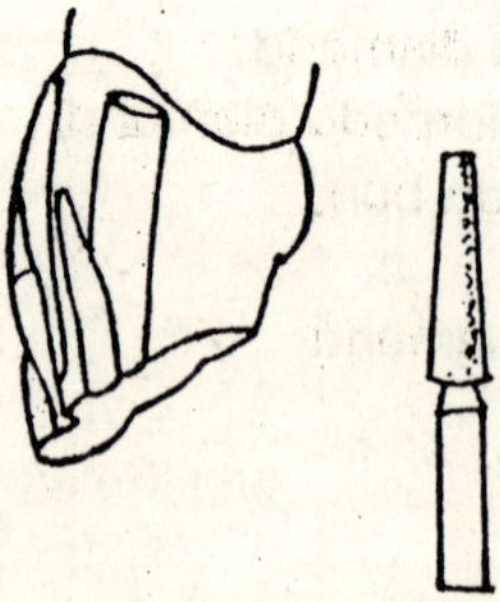

Fig.(5) -Incisal reduction : ***Flat end tapered diamond***

Labial Reduction : This is done in two halves. The incisal half of the labial surface and the cervical half of the labial surface. The incisal half of the labial surface is reduced using a flat end tapered diamond. The bur is held parallel to the incisal half of the labial surface and the tooth substance in between the groove is removed. Using the same bur the cervical half of the labial surface is reduced holding the bur parallel to that surface. Thus the reduction of iabial surface is achieved in two planes. As the bur reduces the labial surface the tip forms the shoulder.

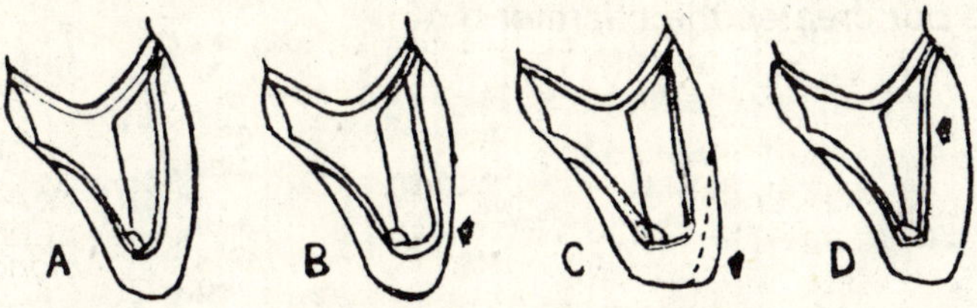

fig (6) - (A) It is important to reduce the labial surface in two planes to receive a porcelain fused to metal restoration (B) if only one plane is produced, opaque porcelain may show through (C) The labial surface only over contoured (D) The pulp may be encroached upon.

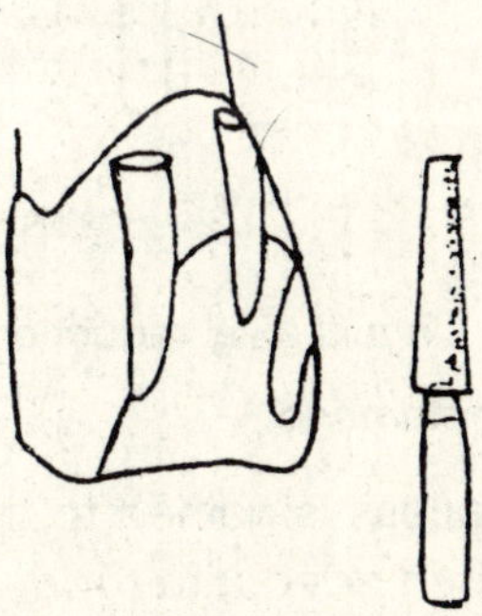

fig (7)- Labial reduction (Incisal half) : *Flat end tapered diamond*

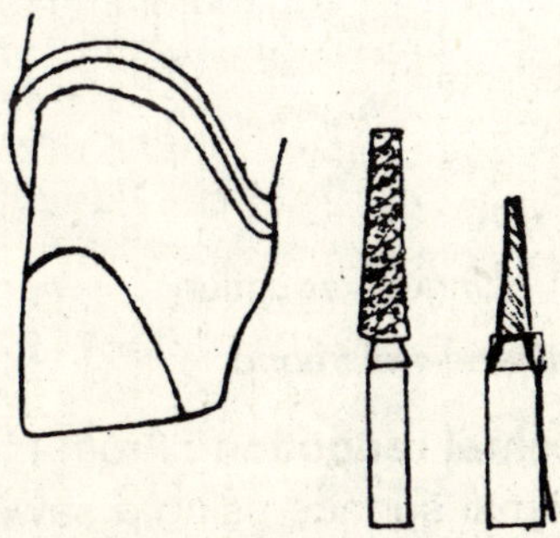

fig(8) - Labial reduction (gingival half) : *Flat end tapered diamond and No. 170 bur*

The reduction is carried out labioproximally to create a wing on either side. The labial surface is smoothened with No. 170 bur. A small bevel may be added to the shoulder later but it is not mandatory.

Lingual Reduction : The lingual reduction is done in two halves. The lingual and the linguoaxial reduction. The lingual reduction is done with a small wheel diamond to obtain a clearance of 0.7mm to 1mm with the opposing teeth. Over shortening the junction between the cingulam and the lingual wall will result in loss of retention. The linguoaxial reduction is done with the chamfer diamond parallel to the gingival portion of the labial surface. The tip of the bur creates the chamfer margin.

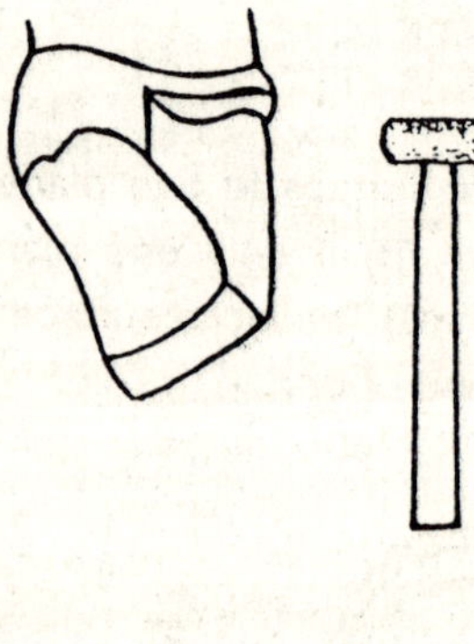

fig(9) - Lingual reduction :
Small wheel diamond

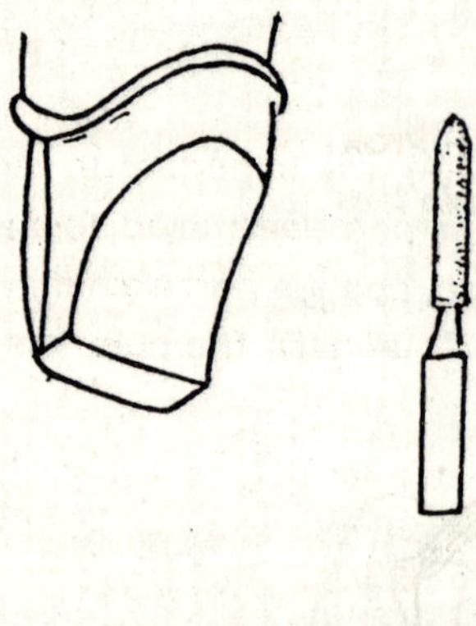

fig.(10)- Lingual axial reduction :
Chamfer diamond

Proximal reduction : From the labial wing access is gained to the proximal surface using a sawing motion. When adequate room is obtained the proximal wall is planed with a chamfer diamond . The bur is held parallel to the long axis of the tooth and the proximal chamfer blends smoothly with the shoulder anteriorly and continues with lingual chamfer posteriorly. The proximal surface and the linguoaxial surface is smoothened with the chamfer bur. The incisal corners are notched with the sides of the chamfer diamond so as to allow the copings to be rounded all over. A narrow bevel (0.2 mm to 0.3mm) may be placed with the tip of the chamfer bur or flame shaped diamond.

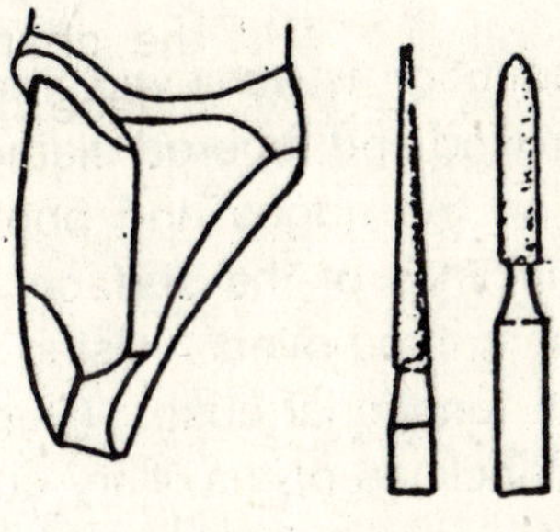

Fig (11)- Proximal axial reduction :
Long thin tapered and chamfer diamond

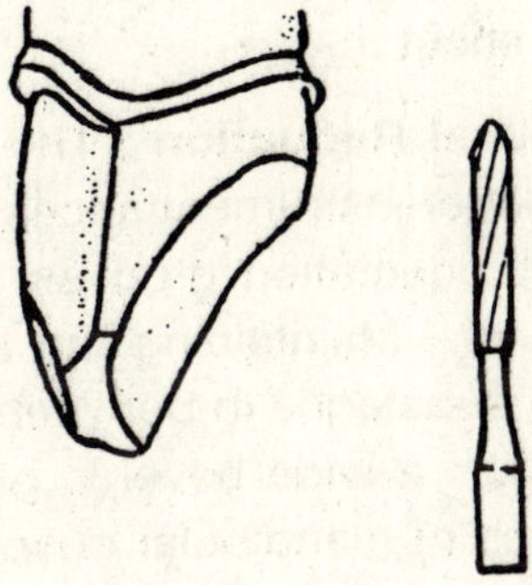

fig (12)- Axial smoothening :
Chamfer bur

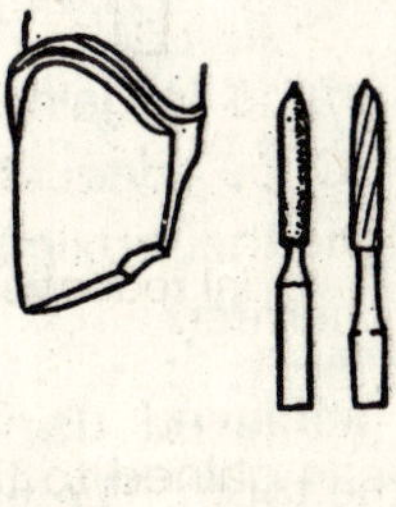

fig (13)- Gingival bevel and incisal ***corners : Chamfer diamond and bur***

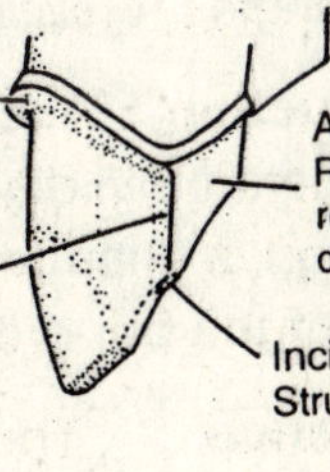

fig (14)- The features of an anterior ***MCR and the function served by each.***

THE POSTERIOR METAL CERAMIC CROWN

Armamentarium

High speed hand piece
Round end tapered diamond and flat end tapered diamond
Chamfer diamond
Rounded wheel
No. 170 bur
Short thin tapered diamond
Wax sheet

Occlusal Reduction : The occlusal reduction is achieved first to get better instrument access. Using a round end tapered diamond depth orientation grooves are placed on the ridges and primary grooves. Maintaining the anatomical inclines of the surface, the tooth substance in between the grooves are removed . Using No. 170 bur a wide bevel is placed on the functional cusp. (Buccal inclines of mandibular cusp and lingual inclines of maxillary cusp) The occlusal clearance is checked with 2 mm thick strip of wax held over the preparation. Insufficient preparation is indicated by a thin spot in the wax. Additional tooth structure in this area is removed and preparation checked with wax sheet again.

Buccal reduction : The buccal wall is reduced with a flat end tapering diamond held parallel to the long axis of tooth. The tip of the bur creates a shoulder. the buccal reduction is carried up to the proximal line angles, creating a wing.

Proximal reduction : Access to the proximal surface is gained using short tapered thin diamond in sawing motion. Once adequate room is obtained, a chamfer diamond is used to plane the proximal walls. The tip of the bur creates the interproximal chamfer.

Lingual reduction : The lingual reduction is achieved using chamfer diamond held parallel to the long axis of the tooth. The tip of the chamfer is used to bevel the buccal shoulder which blends with the interproximal chamfer, which in turn continues with the lingual chamfer.

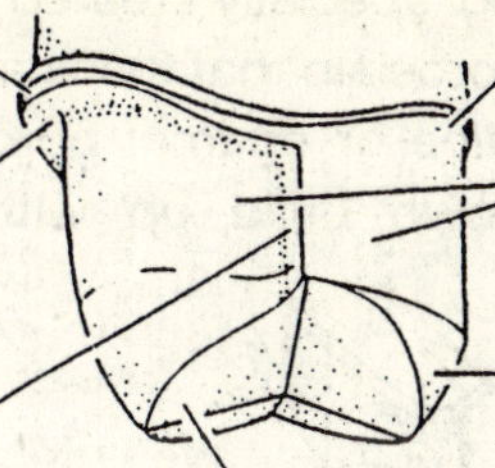

fig (15)- Features of posterior MCR and their functions

COPING DESIGN

There are four important features to be considered when designing the metal coping for MCR :

1. Thickness of metal underlying and adjoining the porcelain.
2. Placement of occlusal and proximal contacts.
3. Extensions of area to be veneered for porcelain.
4. Design of facial margin.

1. Thickness of metal : For adequate strength and rigidity, a noble metal coping should be at least 0.3 to 0.5 mm. A base metal alloy may be as thin as 0.2mm.

2. Occlusal and proximal contacts : Occlusal contact of the opposing teeth should occur on the metal whenever possible. The porcelain metal junction should be 1.0 mm from occlusal contacts at the position of maximum intercusption. see fig.(16)

3. Extent of veneered area : On maxillary molars and premolars the porcelain extends from the buccal surface over the cusp tip about half of the way down the lingual incline of the buccal cusp. The metal over the cusp must be well rounded. When there is a demand for absolute aesthetics the occlusal surface is completely covered with porcelain. The degree of occlusal metal coverage on mandibular molars is dictated by patient's wishes.

4. Facial margin : The present concept is to place an all-porcelain facial margin using specially created shoulder porcelains. These contain aluminous porcelain that fuses at temperature 300°C to 800°C higher than dentine or enamel porcelain. This permits repeated firing of the crown build up with no effect on the completed margin.

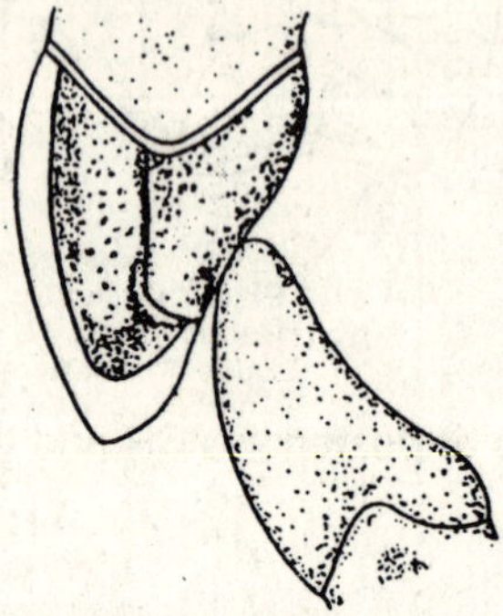

fig. (16) Metal occlusal contact on the lingual surface of maxillary incisors

THE WAX PATTERN FOR MCR

The wax pattern for MCR should be made to the contour of a finished restoration. Then the areas to be veneered are cut back. Only by following this method there can be a smooth continuation of lingual and proximal contours between unveneered metal and porcelain.

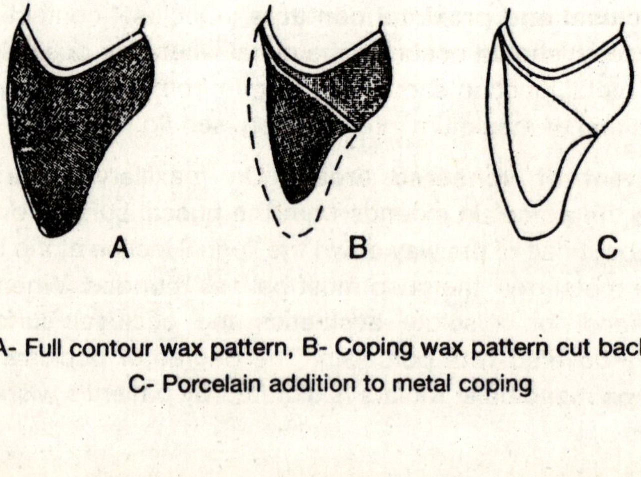

fig.(17) A- Full contour wax pattern, B- Coping wax pattern cut back, C- Porcelain addition to metal coping

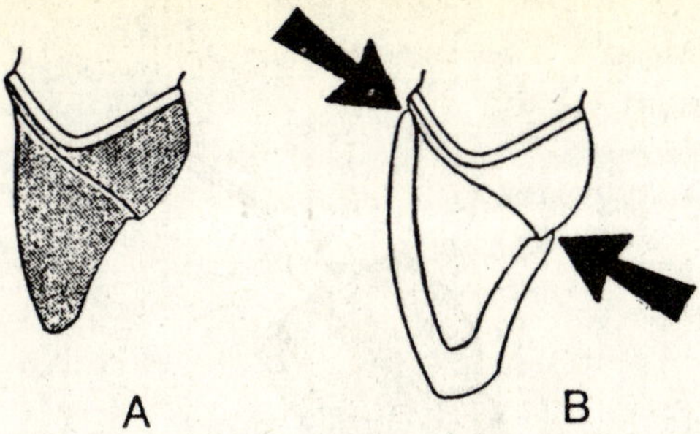

(Fig.18) If the coping pattern (A) is the first step in fabrication, the porcelain veneer on the final restoration may have contours that are not continuous with those of the unveneered coping (B).

ALL WAX TECHNIQUE

Wax is applied on to the lubricated die with a hot spatula. The die is transferred to the working cast to billed axial and proximal contours. Proper occlusal relationship is established. Once the full contour has been established, the pattern is ready to outline the veneering area.

A No.25 blade is used to scratch an outline on the proximal surface of the pattern, as far lingual as possible. Remove 1.5 mm from the incisal portion of an anterior pattern with a knife.

The proximal porcelain metal junction will be approximately 1 mm lingual to the proximal line drawn earlier. Using a discoid carver, orientation grooves are made on the wax pattern, on the labial, mesial and distal surface. From incisal, these grooves must

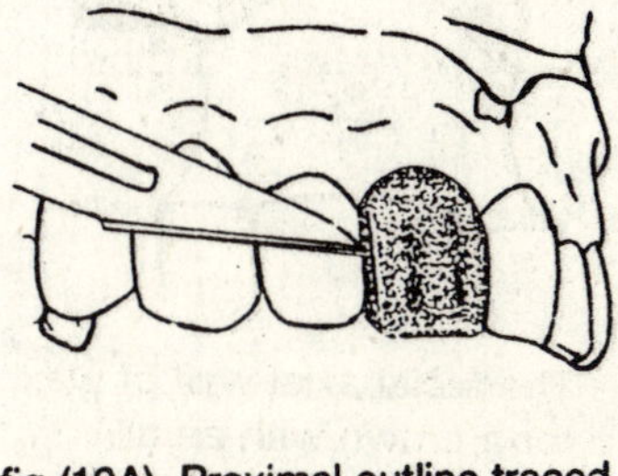

fig (19A) Proximal outline traced with a sharp knife tip

16

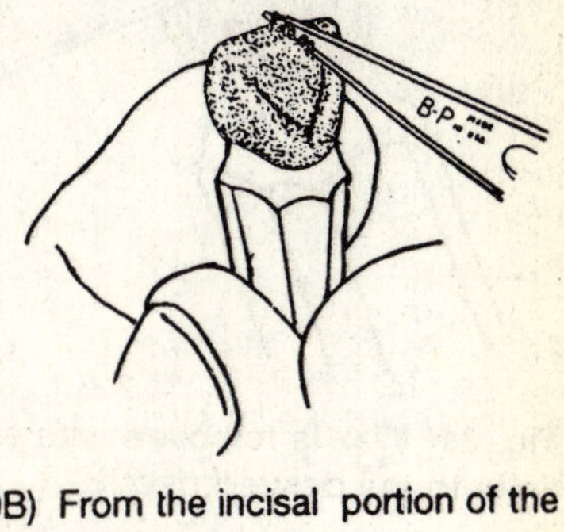

fig (19B) From the incisal portion of the pattern 1.5 mm is cut

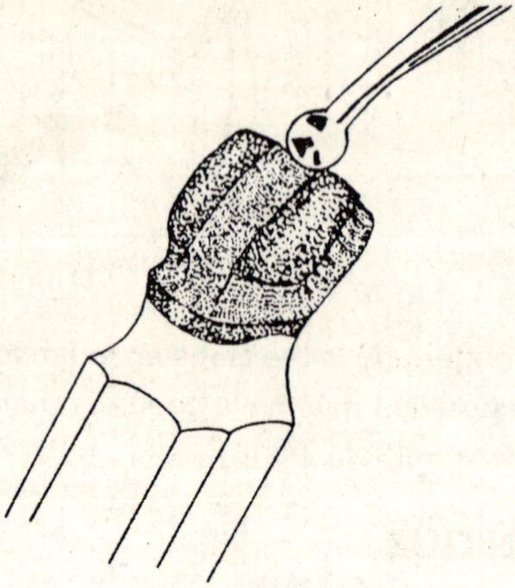

fig.20 Orientation grooves are carved on the wax pattern using a discoid carver.

The design of the facial margin of the restoration is decided before the preparation of tooth itself. For a metal collar, the bulk of wax is removed with knife, leaving behind a collar wax 1 mm wide. The collar will be narrowed approximately 0.3 mm in metal. For an all porcelain facial margin, the wax pattern terminates at the junction of facial axial wall and facial shoulder. The margins are adapted with a beavertail burnisher.

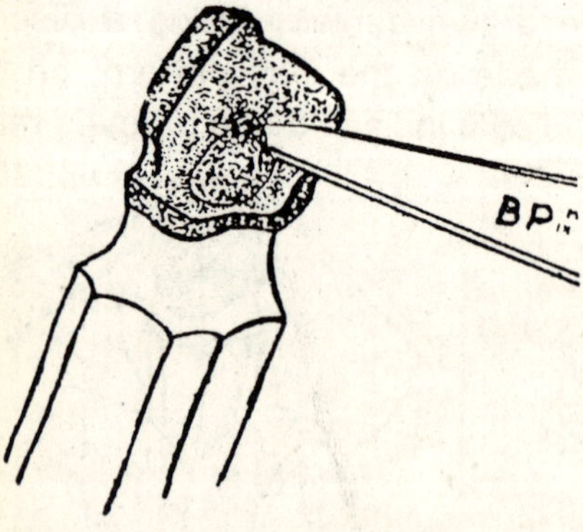

Fig. 21- Wax is removed with sharp knife to the desired depth.

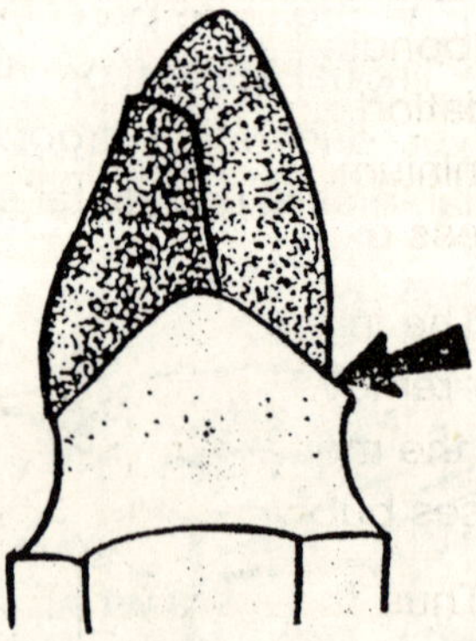

fig.22 - The facial axial wall of wax pattern for a crown with an all porcelain shoulder ends at the gingivo facial angle.

It is better to check the thickness of the wax pattern at this stage. It should be 0.4 - 0.5 mm thick in veneering area. It will be thinned to about 0.3 mm after it has been cast. If it is made too thin at this point it may not cast completely.

ALLOY SURFACE TREATMENT

To enhance the bonding of porcelain to metal, the coping is to be finished with new, clean burs and noncontaminating stones. Aluminium oxide stones and disks should be used in veneering areas. The demarcation line between the veneered and unveneered areas of the coping should be distinct, with an external angle of 90° and a rounded internal angle. The thickness of metal is checked with thickness gauge. Noble metal castings should measure 0.3 mm atleast and base metal castings should measure 0.2 mm. If there is a cervical metal collar, it is narrowed to 0.3 mm. Polishing stones should not be used. Now the coping is ready to undergo oxidation cycle.

Metal surface treatment is unique for each alloy and it is better to follow manufacturer's instructions. Typically, a coping is placed in a furnace at relatively low temperature and the temperature is raised 300° to 400° C at a designated rate of climb.

Heat treatment of noble metal alloys, causes trace elements such as indium and tin in the alloy to form oxides, which enhances the bonding with porcelain. Base metal alloys readily oxidize and oxidation requires control. Following oxidation, air abrasion with aluminium oxide is required to reduce the layer of oxide, since excess oxide weakens the metal ceramic bond.

The initial firing not only causes oxidation of metal surface but also removes the hydrogen from the metal which is incorporated into the molten alloy during firing. If this hydrogen is left behind, it causes bubbles in porcelain, weakening the metal ceramic bond.

Thus the oxidation cycle causes deposition of oxide layer on the metal surface and performs alloy degassing, both of which contributes to bond strength.

Brief description of porcelain build up

Opaque porcelain application

The coping is now ready for porcelain application. It is first painted with a thin coating of distilled water or specially formulated liquid. A small amount of opaque powder is mixed with distilled water or specially formulated liquid forming a thin wash, which is applied with the brush.

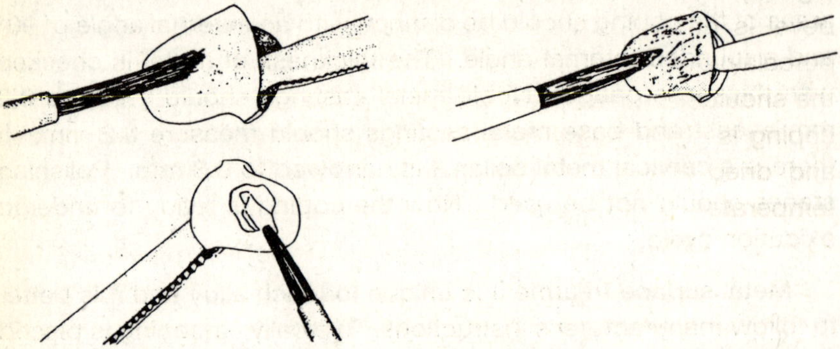

fig. (23) Coping wetted with distilled water.

fig. (24) Thin "Wash" layer is applied with a brush.

At this stage no attempt should be made to completely mask the metal with the first layer of opaque porcelain. The coping is dried and fired under vaccum to specific temperature. The vaccum is broken and coping is held under air for one minute. The second application of opaque porcelain should mask the metal. The powder and liquid are mixed to a creamy consistency and applied to the coping with a brush in a vibrating motion. The opaque layer should be applied as thin as possible. The coping is gently vibrated to condense the porcelain and excess water is removed with dry tissue. The second layer of opaque is fired using the same firing cycle. It must be approximately 0.3 mm thick.

ALL PORCELAIN MARGIN FABRICATION - DIRECT LIFT PORCELAIN MARGIN

The shoulder finish line on the die is marked using the side of a red pencil (fig. 26). The porous surface of gypsum die is sealed using special sealing material. The excess is blown off. A porcelain release agent is applied to the facial shoulder of the sealed die with a brush (fig. 27). The coping is seated on the die. Shoulder porcelain is mixed with distilled water or special liquid and the initial increment is applied to extend 2 to 3 mm on to the metal coping (fig. 28). The porcelain is condensed with the dry tissue. A slight bevel is produced to allow space for a narrow layer of dentine porcelain over shoulder porcelain. Using a sable condensing brush the shoulder porcelain is smoothened at the margin (fig. 29). The coping is gently teased off from the die, placed on a sagger tray and dried in front of the furnace (fig.30). It is then fired at a temperature 30°C higher than the corresponding body porcelain.

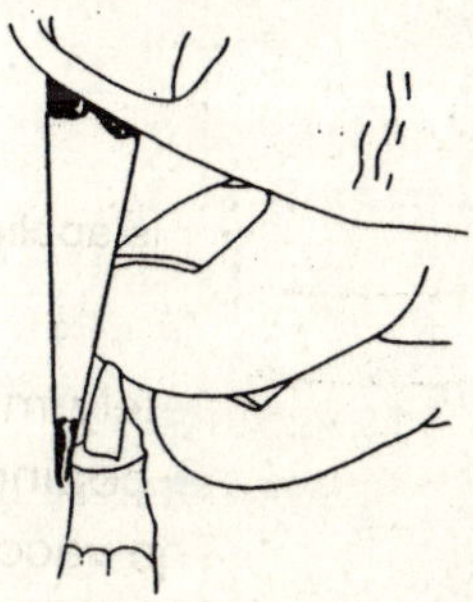

fig. (26) The facial shoulder finish line is marked with the side of a red pencil

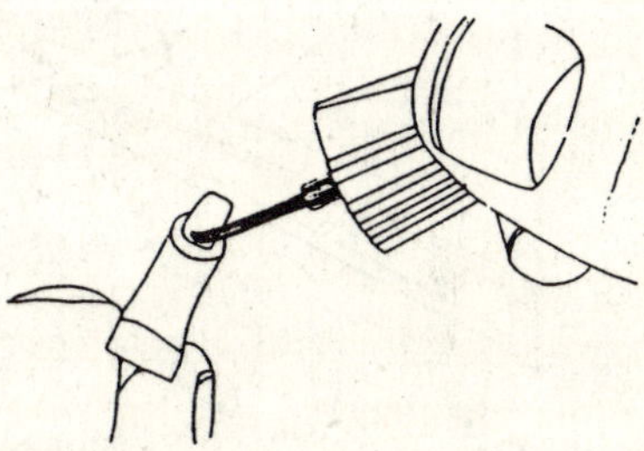

fig. (27) Porcelain release agent is applied to the die around the facial shoulder to prevent porcelain from sticking to the die

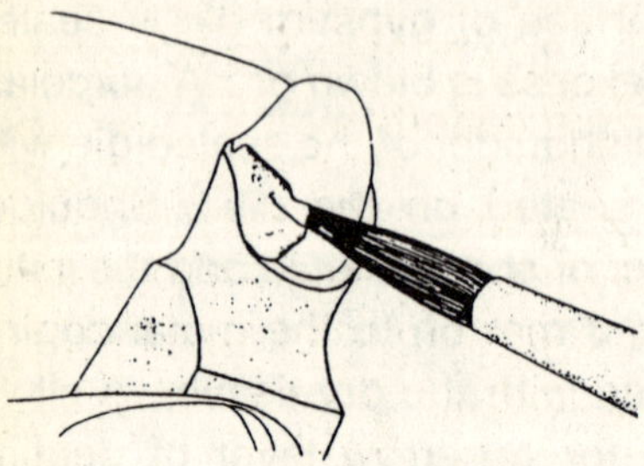

Fig. (28) The shoulder porcelain is applied to the facial shoulder of the die with a brush It should extend 2-3 mm on to the metal coping

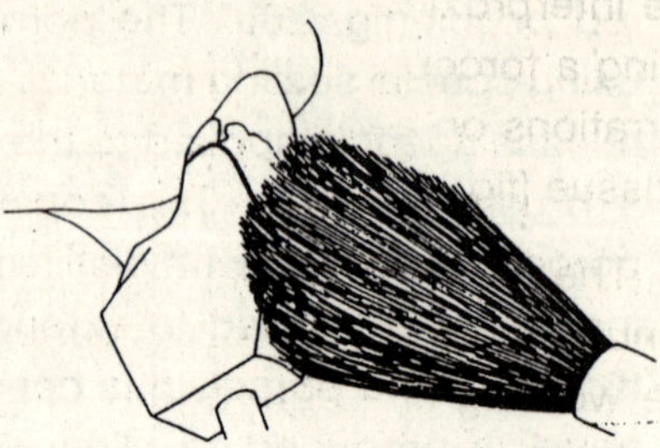

fig. (29) A large no.10 sable brush is used to smooth the margin and remove excess bulk.

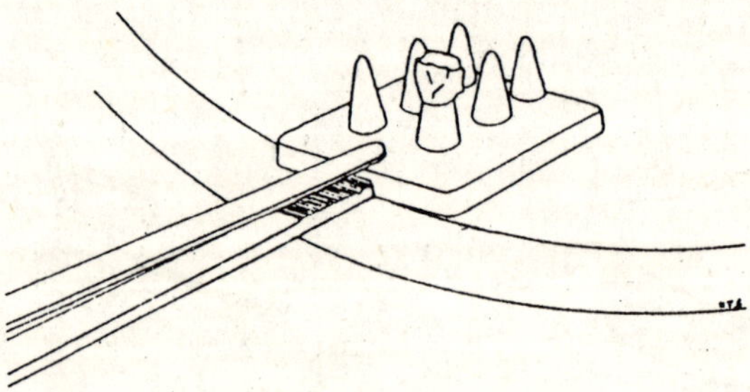

fig. (30) The coping is placed on a sagger tray and dried in front of the oven door.

Dentine And Enamel Porcelain Application

The dentine porcelain is mixed with dístilled water and applied on the opaque to obtain full contour of the tooth. The tissue is held behind the incisal edge [fig. 31].The build-up is over contoured, to a size one fifth larger than the desired length. It is dried to get wet sand consistency. Then the denture porcelain is carved back to allow the placement of enamel porcelain. The amount cut back will decide the degree of translucency [fig. 32]. The restoration is carefully removed from the working cast and porcelain is added to the interproximal area [fig. 33]. The crown is removed off the die using a forceps. It is condensed by vibrating the forceps with the serrations on a roach carver. The surface moisture is blotted using a tissue [fig. 34].

The initial build-up is dried in front of the furnace for several minutes and then fired under vaccum. The restoration is tried on the working cast and all contours evaluated [fig. 35]. Insufficient contours are corrected by adding appropriate porcelain and fired at temperatures 10°C-20°C lower than initial bake. Following correction bake, the crown may not seat completely. Adjustments are made with aluminium oxide stones and discs.

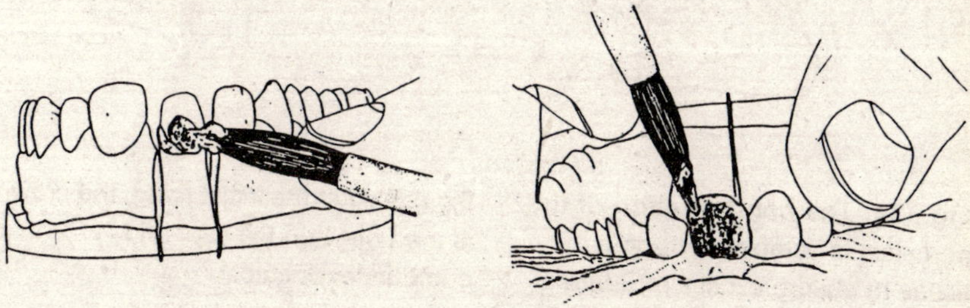

Fig (31) Build up of the detine porcelain is continued with the brush while holding a piece of tissue behind the incisal edge to absorb water.

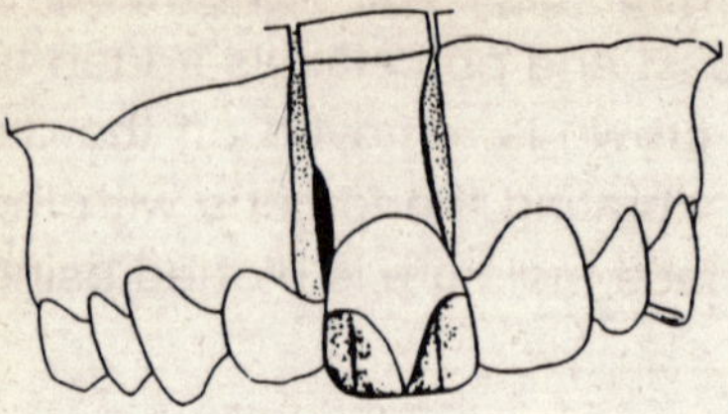

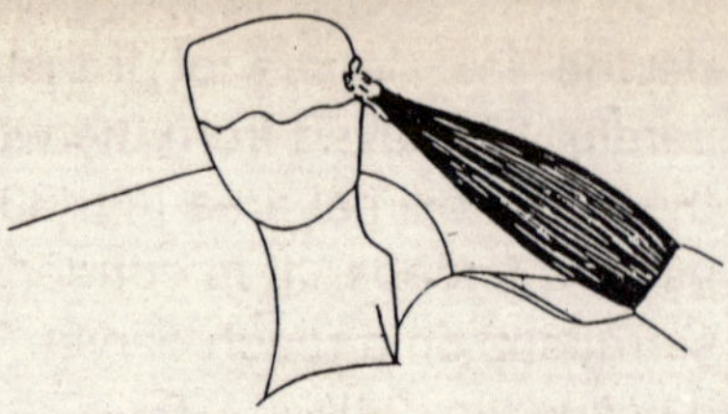

Fig. (32) Completion of cutback for the incisal porcelain.

Fig (33) The die is removed from the cast and a small amount of porcelain is added to the two interproximal surfaces.

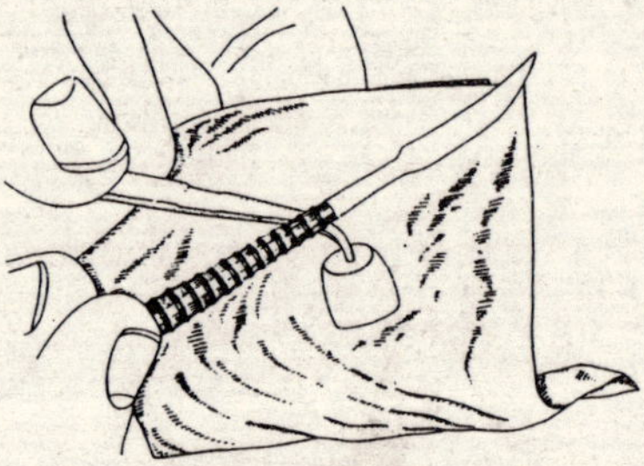

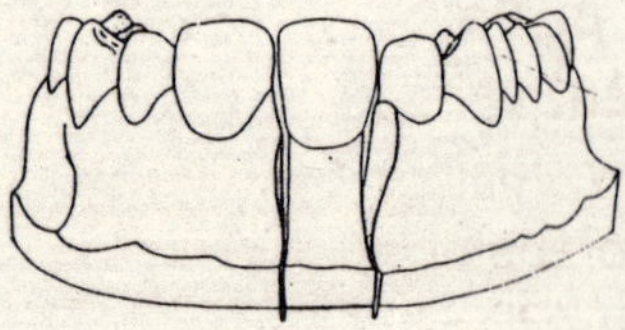

Fig. (34) The condensation of the porcelain is completed using a tissue to absorb excess moisture

Fig (35) After the initial firing, the crown is tried back on the cast and contours evaluated.

PORCELAIN SURFACE TREATMENT

Completed porcelain restoration may be treated by :

1) Auto glaze,

2) Over glaze, or

3) Polishing.

Rubberised abrasives and polishing compounds are available to polish porcelain.

1. Auto Glaze : Porcelain has the ability to glaze itself when held at its fusing temperature under air for 1 to 4 minutes.

2. Over Glaze : Applied over glaze is a low fusing clear porcelain that is painted on the surface of the restoration and fired at a temperature much lower than the fusion temperature of dentine and enamel porcelain. Porcelain normally loses its ability to form natural glaze after multiple firing. An applied over glaze is indicated for large restorations that have required number of corrections. At this point it must be understood that if devitrification of porcelain occurs, no amount of surface treatment will revive the natural appearance of porcelain.

3. Polished Porcelain : Traditionally polished porcelain has been regarded to have a rougher surface than glazed porcelain. Low fusing porcelains are highly polishable in the mouth decreasing the need for glazing procedure after intra oral corrections.

The metal ceramic restoration indeed forms the crowning glory of restorative dental practice. Not only they are widely used as extra coronal restorations, but they find a place in intra coronal restorations too. Resin bonded metal ceramic inlays have been used, where aesthetic demands are high. The tooth preparation is similar to the standard gold inlay restorations. A heavy gingival chamfer is given and occlusaly the cavity margin should be formed at an obtuse angle. The minimal depth of cavity should be 2.5 mm. Vertical retention grooves may be formed on the proximal box to provide resistance against lateral forces. The only disadvantage of this procedure is additional laboratory expertise necessary to fabricate the restoration.

A more recent, major modification of one of the system is digital scanning of gypsum die. Once the data is loaded, the system software can manipulate the scanned image to define the preparation finish line, coping thickness and cervical collar design and also the space for luting agent. The data can be transferred by modem to a remote manufacturer for production of titanium fixed prosthesis frame work. Metal ceramic crowns based on swaged foil copings have been designed to fabricate the metal coping without casting process (fig. 36)

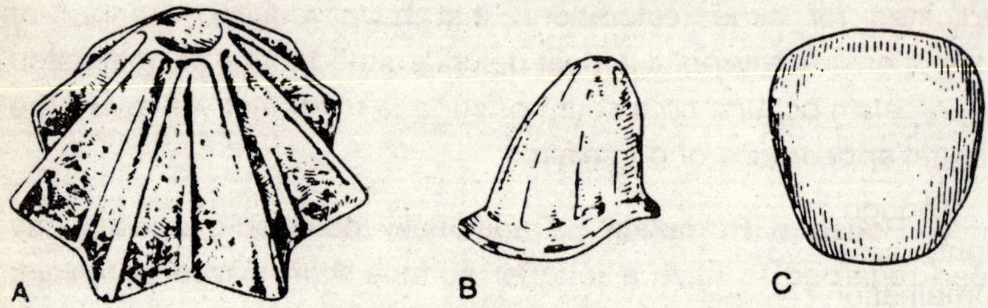

(fig. 36)

The pleated gold foil is swaged over the die with a swaging instrument, burnished with hand instrument and then flame sintered (fig. 37) to form coping with moderate strength. An interfacial alloy powder is applied and fired. The coping is then veneered with porcelain. The most outstanding advantage of the metal ceramic restoration is its aesthetic quality and strength. Occlusal surfaces can be boldly veneered with low fusing porcelains since their ability to abrade the opposing natural tooth is very minimal. The fracture rates of metal ceramic crown as well as bridges is 2.3% after 7.5 years. The metal ceramic restorations which produces unsurpassed cosmetic results is today well within the reach of every practicing dentist. It is, and will remain the crowning glory of restorative dental practice.

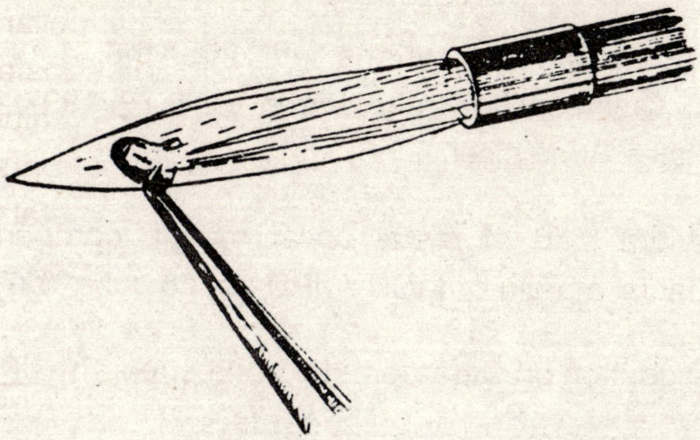

(fig. 37)

Though a number of newer restorative materials, which are highly aesthetically pleasing are being developed, the bonded combination of metal and ceramics still reign supreme.

REFERENCES

1. Phillip's Science of Dental Materials - Anusavice
2. Contemporary Fixed Prosthodontics - Stephen F. Rosenstiel
3. Ceramo metal Fixed Partial Dentures - George Isaacson, Daniel Isaacson.
4. Retention and resistance of preparation of cast restorations Potts R.G. Shillingburg HT. JPD 43:303-308 : March 1980.
5. Preparation design and margin distortion in porcelain fused to metal restoration - JPD, 29:276-284, March 1973.
6. Principles of Tooth preparation - H.T. Shillingburg Jacobi

7. A new metal Ceramic Crown - JPD 40:273, 1978. Mc Lean J.W., Bruggers. H.

8. Esthetic posterior restorations utilizing, the double-inlay technique - Quintessence International 2.28L79, 1997. Mathias Hanning Raine Schmeiser.

9. In vitro failure load of metal collar margin compared with porcelain facial margin of MCR - JPD Vol 78 July 1997.

10. Effect of Oxidation on Ceramometal bond strength - JPD 1982, 47:5962.

11. Phillips RW. Skinners Science of Dental Material - ed. 9: WB Sauders Co. 1991 P.505-527.

LUTING CEMENTS

Balagopal S.

Luting cement is used for attaching fabrications which may be made of metal, resin, ceramic, metal with resin or metal with ceramic to the tooth surface. A luting cement may be used for any of the following reasons :

1) To give a provisional restoration for a short period such as few days. For example temporary crowns made of resin or metal in the anterior or posterior teeth, until a ceramic crown or a final restoration is made for the teeth.

2) To cement a restoration for a longer period such as few weeks to months. Such interim restorations are given for a tooth under doubtful prognosis, when a permanent restoration can be planned only after a longer period, and for cementing orthodontic appliances.

3) Permanent cementation that requires the restoration to be in place for longest period of time possible. Inlays, Onlays, Crowns, Bridges and Laminates all require such long-term durability.

The function of traditional luting cement is to provide retention by interlocking between the minor irregularities on both the prepared tooth surface and the restoration surface. The narrower the cement lute, the stronger the bond and the better the marginal fit of the restoration, the longer the cement lute will last. The newer adhesive cements with polyacrylic acid and those with complex organic chemicals in resin based luting agents claim to have true chemical union to the tooth surface or restoration surface or both. Though achieving a chemical bonding is the ultimate goal, as of now it does not appear to have radically altered the concept of the original retentive role of the luting cements.

REQUIREMENTS:

Luting cements should have low solubility in oral fluids as well as in dietary chemicals. Adhesion to tooth structure is an additional advantageous property. Adhesion of the cement to tooth surface will reduce or eliminate microleakage between the tooth and the restoration and thus prevent the consequent tooth sensitivity and secondary caries.

Fluoride leach and anti-cariogenic property would also be very beneficial.

Luting cement must be sufficiently fluid and be able to flow into a continuous film of 25μ thickness or less. The lower the viscosity of the material the better its wetting ability and greater its adaptability. That is why for cementation a mix with lowest viscosity, which can be biologically and mechanically acceptable, should be used. This means that the important physical property of a luting cement is its compressive and shear strength.

It should be biocompatible. In a freshly prepared tooth, the dentinal tubules are wide open and the pulp would become hyperemic due to the trauma of cutting as well. In such cases the irritant cement would have a profound effect upon the pulp. Hence the luting cement should be kind to pulp and help heal inflamed pulp tissue as well.

PROCEDURE FOR CEMENTATION:

The cement paste should be coated on the entire fitting surface of the restoration. A little excess should be present in the margins and flow beyond the margin. In the case of crowns the cement should fill half the space of the fitting surface volume. This is necessary to displace the air from the occlusal surface of the crown before the sides of the occlusal surface come in contact with the walls of the crown. The restoration should be immediately seated with care to prevent entrapment of air. After ensuring that the path of insertion is also right, a continuous increase in pressure is applied over the restoration to displace the excess cement and move the restoration as close to fitting as possible. Vibration instruments may also be used for this. The marginal fit is then inspected. Making the patient bite on a piece of softwood, rubber or biting device completes the seating. This pressure should be sustained till the initial setting of the cement is complete.

REMOVAL OF EXCESS CEMENT:

The excess cement is removed by force exerted along the direction of the seating of the restoration, which is usually in a apical direction. A sharp instrument is used with a deft stroke to break the mass from outside the margin of the restoration. Dental floss with a knot tied in it is quite effective in removing cement from the interproximal area. Any cement left in the gingival crevices will be highly irritant to the gingiva as well as unpleasant for the patient.

The time of removal of the excess cement depends on the properties of the cements used -

1) If the cement sets to a brittle state and does not adhere to the surrounding surfaces, the tooth and the restoration, it is best removed after it sets. Examples are ZPC, SPC and ZOE

2) For those cements that are capable of adhering to the surrounding tissues both physical or chemical, the excess cements may be removed by one of the following methods -

Adjacent surfaces to the filling area may be coated with a separating media such as cocoa butter or petroleum jelly. This inhibits the adherence of the cements to these surfaces. Then once the cement sets hard to a brittle state it can be broken away.

The excess cement extruding out should be removed immediately after seating the restoration preventing the material from adhering to the adjacent surfaces.

CAUTION:

The cement should not be removed when it is in a rubbery stage, as it is turning into a brittle solid. If attempted, the cement from the marginal area may be pulled out resulting in a gap between the restoration and the tooth surface.

POST CEMENTATION:

1. Aqueous based cements continue to mature over time. During this period it has to be protected. Contamination with oral fluid will

result in washing away of the immature cement from the margin. Some cement loses water during the setting process if exposed to dry atmosphere. This would make the cement porous and easily soluble in oral fluid on setting. Hence to allow the cement to mature in an isolated environment the margins of the restoration may be coated with varnish, lacquer or proprietary protective.

2. Resin cements set chemically under anaerobic environment. If exposed to atmospheric air, the margins of the cements do not polymerize completely. As a result the cement in the margin becomes weak, easily imbibes (sorbs) water, leaches out unused monomer to surrounding tissues as well as undergoes discoloration. The margins of the restoration have to be protected using proprietary gels or deoxigeniser.

3. Damage to the cement at the margin of the restoration results in leakage or plaque accumulation and produces sensitivity and secondary caries.

Like cements used for restorations, luting cements may also be classified according to their chemical composition. The cements that are good luting agents are Zinc Phosphate, Zinc Copper Phosphate, Zinc silicophosphate, Glass longmer cements, Poly Carboxylate cements, Zinc Oxide Eugenol [ZOE] Cements, and Resin cements.

ZINC SILICOPHOSPHATE CEMENT:

This is a hybrid cement from the combination of zinc phosphate cement and silicate cement which has been in use since 1878. It is also known by the names zinc silicate cements, silicate zinc cements and most popularly as just silicophosphate cements.

Dispensing:

The cement is dispensed as a powder and a liquid.

Some common brands marketed are - 'Fluoro-Thin'; 'Petralit'; and 'Kryptex'

Composition:

The powder contains high percentage of acid soluble silicate with varying amounts of zinc and magnesium oxides. The liquid is an aqueous solution of phosphoric acid with zinc and aluminum salts added as a buffer.

The composition of one of the proprietary cements is

POWDER

Silica	35%
Alumina	25%
Zinc oxide	10% - 20%
Fluorides of Calcium and Sodium	17%
Calcium oxide or lime	1% - 5%

LIQUID

Phosphoric acid	48%
Water	35%
Buffers	17%

Types:

This cement is available in the following types -

Type I	Used as a luting agent
Type II	Used for temporary restoration of posterior teeth
Type III	Used for dual purpose

Setting Reaction:

Zinc Aluminosilicate glass + Phosphoric acid = Zinc Alumino silico phosphate gel.

The setting reaction produces a matrix of zinc and alumnium phosphate enclosing unreacted core of zinc oxide and glass particles.

Manipulation:

Proportioning:

Powder liquid ratio: As much powder as possible should be incorporated into the mix while maintaining the consistency.

Mixing:

The powder is divided into two equal parts. One half is divided into three to four parts to adjust consistency.

The first half of the powder is incorporated into two to three drops of liquid and then smaller parts are added as mixing proceeds. Mixing is done by folding, tapping and overlapping technique. The mix has a putty consistency. The total mixing time should not exceed one minute.

The Effect of Mixing Method, Humidity and Slab Temperature on the Cement:

As the temperature of the mixing slab decreases the powder liquid ratio necessary to achieve a standard consistency increases. Working time on the mixing slab increases as the mixing temperature is lowered. Setting time in the oral environment decreases when the cement is mixed at decreased temperatures. At reduced temperature the rate of incorporation of powder had no effect on any of the properties but at room temperature rapid incorporation results in less than optimum properties. Moisture free mixes at reduced temperatures result in higher compressive and tensile strengths for the cements. Setting time of the cement is 3.5 to 4 minutes

Mechanical Properties:

Compressive strength	- 130 - 175 MN/m^2 (145MPa) (19,900 - 25000psi)
Diametrical tensile strength	- 7.6 MPa (1100psi)
Solubility and disintegration in water	- 0.4% weight
Film Thickness	- upto 88μ

The mechanical properties are somewhat higher than zinc phosphate cements. It is relatively stiff and should have a modulus of elasticity in the range of zinc phosphate cements (1.3 - 1.9 x 10^6 psi)

Silicophosphate cements are translucent and hence they are superior to zinc phosphate for cementation of ceramic restorations. The stiffness suggests its applicability as a luting agent for ceramic restorations, where they are subjected to functional loads. Since the type I cement is recommended for the cementation of precision casting it should meet a maximum film thickness of 25μm. Although the film thickness is slightly greater than 25μm, it is preferred for the cementation of porcelain restoration due to its translucency. A small space created by the removal of platinum matrix from the porcelain restoration fabricated by conventional techniques made the film thickness in these cases less critical. It is not generally used for the cementation of the precision casting. However recent formulations with decreased film thickness and improved handling characteristics are available for the cementation of gold and precision castings.

Biological Properties:

Silico phosphate cement is very irritant to the pulp. The pH remains lower than 3 for more than 30minutes after cementing. The pH remains low for few days. Hence a cavity varnish is applied before the cementation with this material, due to its acidity. Zinc silico phosphate is less soluble in the mouth than zinc phosphate. These cements inhibit secondary caries due to the release of fluorides from the silicate component of the powder. Hence it has anticariogenic potential.

ZINC OXIDE EUGENOL CEMENT [ZOE]

Zinc oxide eugenol cement has been extensively used in dentistry since the 1890ís. It has a sedative effect on the pulp and is specially useful for cementation on prepared teeth with freshly cut and exposed dentinal tubules. The addition of reenforcing agents to ZnO has resulted in permonent luting cement. Hence for luting there is a type one ZnO cement used for temporary cementation and a type II material used for permanent cementation. Temporary luting cement (Type I) is not as strong as Type II permanent luting cement. It is useful for short-term cementation of temporaries. Non eugenol zinc oxide cement is also available as a luting agent. It is particularly useful in cementing acrylic temporaries which otherwise are chemically attacked by the eugenol in the regular cement.

Dispensing:

Dispensed as powder and Liquid.

Some common brands are- Polymer based- 'Fynal', 'Staline'. Alumina EBA based - 'Opotow'

Composition:

a. Unmodified

Powder:

Zinc oxide	69% by weight
White rosin	29.3%
Zinc stearate	1%
Zinc acetate	1%

Liquid:

Eugenol	85%
Olive oil	15%

b. EBA cement:

The powder contains zinc oxide 65% -75%, quartz 20 - 35%, hydrogenated rosin 5% and the pink colored liquid contains about 62.5% orthoethoxy benzoic acid and 37.5% eugenol.

Types:

TYPE I - Temporary cementation.

TYPE II - Permanent cementation of restorations

TYPE III - Temporary filling material and thermal insulating base

TYPE IV - Liner

Setting Reaction:

It is basically an Acid - Base reaction

Zinc Oxide + Water = Zinc Hydroxide

Zinc Hydroxide + Eugenolic Acid = Zinc Eugenolate + Water.

Reaction takes place either in solution or at the surface of zinc oxide particles. The water that is formed in the setting reaction probably aids in binding the individual chelate units together, possibly in a chain or in an octahedral structure or it may be merely absorbed by the excess zinc oxide. The first reaction consist of hydrolysis of zinc oxide to its hydroxide indicating that water is essential for the reaction. The reaction is autocatalytic. Dehydrated zinc oxide will not react with dehydrated eugenol. The chelate is thought to form an amorphous mass that tends to crystallize, imparting increased strength to the set mass. Formation of crystalline zinc eugenolate is greatly enhanced when the setting reaction is accelerated by zinc dehydrate, which is more soluble than zinc hydroxide and thus can supply zinc ions more rapidly

Manipulation:

Proportioning:

Powder liquid ratio is 4.5 gms of powder per ml. of eugenol.

Mixing procedure:

Cement intended for luting should follow the manufacturer's direction and measuring devices, because of the deceptive flow qualities of these cements. Adding powder until the operator feels the mix is of suitable consistency for cementation will lead to cement deficient in powder and a lowered strength. A cool mixing slab is not required, as the setting reaction is not exothermic. A glass slab and a stiff bladed steel spatula are used. There is no need to incorporate the powder in small increments and usually the bulk of the powder is incorporated in the initial step. The mix is thoroughly spatulated and then a series of smaller amounts are added till the mix is complete. The mix is thoroughly kneaded with a spatula. Mixing time is about 90 seconds.

The EBA cements are dispensed according to the instructions. After incorporating the powder into the liquid, the mass is kneaded for 30 seconds and then stropped for 60 seconds with broad strokes of the spatula to develop a creamy consistency. This cement can set to a very hard mass and adhere to surrounding tissues and external surface of the restoration. Oil of orange is a solvent used to remove the set cement.

Properties:

I. Compressive Strength

A maximum value of 35MN/m^2 is required for cement intended for temporary cementing and a minimum of 35MN/m^2 is required for permanent cementing. Type I cement has a compressive strength of 6 - 28 MN/m^2 and Type II cement with ZOE + Alumina + EBA 55 MN/m^2 and Type II cement with ZOE and polymer 48 MN/m^2.

2. Setting Shrinkage

ZOE exhibits the least amount of shrinkage of all the materials. This is only 0.1% of the volume.

3. Coefficient of Thermal Expansion

It has a coefficient of thermal expansion that is closest to that of tooth structure, which is about 11ppm/1°C.

4. Solubility and Disintegration

A maximum value of 2.5% is acceptable. It is measured by weight loss that occurs in a disc of cement immersed in distilled water for 24hours.

5. Flow:

Unmodified ZOE has the highest flow among all the cements. In ZOE the flow is increased by increasing the P/L ratio and by the addition of fillers, rosin and EBA. Flow can also be increased by increasing the shearing energy induced during manipulation. Increasing the temperature also increases the flow of the cement due to the thermoplastic nature of ZOE.

6. Film Thickness

The Film thickness of ZOE is about 25 - 35µm.

7. Viscosity

Viscosity is directly proportional to the P/L ratio, temperature, particle size and inversely proportional to the energy used in mixing and inserting. ZOE has a moderate viscosity.

Biocompatibility with Pulp-Dentin Organ:

ZOE has a pH of 7 and hence is least irritating to the PD organ. ZOE does not increase the penetrability of the underlying dentin. On the contrary with its multiple pharmacological actions such as sedation to pulp, healing of inflamed pulp, anodyne effect it can also enhance the sclerosing of the underlying dentin. It has a low thermal diffusivity and can also provide electrical insulation.

Temporary Cementation

Type I cements:

The unmodified ZOE is used as luting material for temporary crowns and temporary cementation of gold restorations and in crown and Bridge prosthodontics. Retention of these restorations is proportional to the compressive strength of the cements. Cement with a compressive strength from 2200 - 3500 psi [15.2 - 24.1MN/m^2] was the most appropriate on the basis of retention, ease of removal and ease of cleaning. Type I ZOE meets these requirements. It seals the cavity well against the ingress of fluids. Hence irritation caused by microleakage is minimized during the period of temporization.

The non-eugenol cement does not adhere well to metal crowns as does the eugenol containing cement. It is also slower in setting. The non-eugenol cement however does not soften temporary resin crowns and hence are very useful.

Permanent Cementation

Type II ZOE cement or modified ZOE cement is used for luting permanent restorations as it has increased compressive strength and decreased solubility. EBA encourages the formation of a crystalline structure, which imparts greater strength to the set material. Compressive strength of this cement is increased upto 60 MPa. There is lower level of residual eugenol coupled with greater resistance to hydrolysis of zinc-ortho-ethoxybenoate that produces cement with a lower solubility.

Cement has been developed containing hexyl vanalate as a substitute for eugenol. It has been claimed that this cement has increased strength and lesser solubility than EBA modified cement.

Disadvantages of modified ZOE cement is that the mechanical properties are inferior to other cements. It is somewhat difficult to manipulate in the oral cavity and the film thickness tends to be high and the set cement excess is difficult to remove. For these reasons type II ZOE cement is confined primarily to those situations in which anticipated sensitivity might be a problem.

ZINC PHOSPHATE CEMENT

This cement was introduced in the year 1878 and is the oldest cement of all those used in Dentistry. It is also known by the names 'Crown and Bridge Cement' and zinc oxy phosphate cement. It can produce the thinnest film thickness of the available cements yet provide the highest compressive strength. The primary and traditional use of this cement is only to lute cast restorations to the teeth. This cement has self etching property which enhances the surface irregularity and adhesion to tooth structure. It was originally adapted from a substance containing zinc chloride used for cementing mosaic tiles to the walls and floors. Later it was modified because zinc chloride is harmful to the pulp.

Dispensing:

They are available as Type I and Type II cements. They are commonly dispensed in bulk as powder and liquid. Some products are supplied pre-encapsulated in syringes. They are also available in few selected shades of yellow and gray.

The Type I cement has finer particle size and is used for seating precision appliances.

The type II cements are the traditionally used cements for all luting purposes.

Some common brands are 'Lee Smith Zinc', 'Pennwalt', 'Fleckís Extraordinary', 'Modern Tinacin', and 'Harvard Zinc Phosphate Cement'.

Composition:

POWDER-

ZO	90.2%
MgO	8.2%
SiO_2	1.4%
$Bi2O_3$	0.1%
Miscellaneous (BaO, Ba_2SO_4, CaO)	0.1%

LIQUID:

Phosphoric acid (free acid)	38.2
Phosphoric acid combined with Alumina and zinc	16.2%
Alumina	2.5%
Zinc	7.1%
Water	36.0%

Powder-

The principal ingredient of ZPC is zinc oxide. Magnesium oxide in quantities of about 10% is added to zinc oxide to reduce the temperature of the calcination process. Although Bismuth oxide is believed to impart a smoothness to a freshly mixed cement mass, in large amounts it may also lengthen the setting time. Some contain tannin fluoride which provides a source of fluoride ions for anticariogenic effect. The ingredients of the powder are heated together at temperatures of about 1000deg to 1300deg centigrade for a prolonged period of time of approximately 4 to 8 hours or longer depending on the temperature employed. This calcination results in a fused or sintered mass. The mass is then ground and pulverised to a fine powder which is sieved to recover selected particle sizes. The degree of calcination, the fineness of the particle size, and the composition determine the reactivity, the powder will have with the liquid.

ZPC powders may be obtained in a variety of colors. The lighter shades of yellow and gray are the most popular and these combined with other yellows, grays, golden browns and pink are advantages for some cementations. A proper blend of shades may decidedly enhance the esthetic qualities of a porcelain restoration. Some shades of cement powder are attained by regulating the amount of calcination the powders receive. But the common method is to develop various shades by the addition of minute quantities of certain pigmenting substances to the ground powders. Copper oxide, Manganese dioxide, platinum black and powdered charcoal have been used to produce various shades of gray. Yellow powders may be produced by the addition of yellow bismuth oxide, certain chromates or organic pigments. Iron oxide or titanium compounds are often used to produce the brown or cream colored powders. Quantities ranging from 1/2000 to 1/5000 parts of cement are sufficient to develop a required shade using these metal oxide pigments.

Liquid-

Zinc phosphate liquid is produced by the addition of aluminum or sometimes zinc or their compounds to an orthophosphric acid solution. Although the original acid solution contains about 85% phosphoric acid and is a syrupy fluid, the resulting cement liquid usually contains about 1/3 water. The partial neutralization of the phosphoric acid by the aluminum and zinc, tempers the reactivity of the liquid and is described as buffering. This reduced rate of reaction aids in establishing a smooth non granular workable cement mass during the mixing procedure. The presence of additional water to phosphoric acid shortens the setting time, whereas insufficient amount of water results in a prolonged setting time. The zinc phosphate cement liquid is therefore adjusted by both partial neutralizing or buffering and dilution so that it will react with its powder to produce a cement mass with proper setting time and mechanical qualities.

Chemistry of Setting Reaction:

When the powder is incorporated into the liquid, a chemical reaction begins. When zinc oxide is mixed with an aqueous solution of phophoric acid, the superficial layer of the zinc oxide is dissolved by the acid. In the case of pure zinc oxide mixed with phosphoric acid, the acid base reaction first involves the formation of an acid phosphate.

$$ZnO + 2H3PO_4 = + Zn(H_2PO_4)_2 + H_2O$$

This is followed by a further reaction where a hydrated zinc phosphate is produced.

$$ZnO + Zn(H_2PO_4)_2 + 2H_2O = Zn_3\ (PO_4)4H_2O[\text{Hopeite}]$$

This substance is virtually insoluble and crystallizes to form a phosphate matrix, which binds together the unreacted parts to the zinc oxide particles. The reaction is slightly exothermic and some shrinkage of cement takes place. It is thought that in the commercial materials the presence of aluminium prevents the crystallization process, producing a glassy matrix in the form of an alumino phosphate gel. This lack of crystallization is exacerbated by the presence of magnesium, which delays the development of any crystals. Some amount of crystallization resulting in the formation of hopeite may occur with time. Unbound water forms globules within the material resulting in a porous structure and makes the cement highly permeable when the material is dry. The final structure is that of particles of unreacted zinc oxide in a matrix consisting of phosphate of zinc, magnesium and aluminium.

Manipulation:

Powder - Liquid Ratio :

The manner in which the reaction between the zinc phosphate cement powder and liquid is permitted to occur determines to a large extent the working characteristics and the properties of the set cement mass. The powder - liquid ratio depends on the application. For luting, a more fluid mix with a lower powder - liquid ratio is employed to ensure a flow of cement during the seating of the restoration. When proportioning it is important to remember that lowering the powder - liquid ratio produces a weaker, more soluble and more irritant material. It is prudent to follow the manufacturer's instructions strictly to get a proper consistency with optimum properties of the cement. The amount of liquid with which the powder is combined to form a sufficient quantity of inlay cement of luting consistency is about 0.25ml. The cement liquid dispensing droppers supplied by the manufacturers may each expel drops that vary in volume slightly from one dropper to another. No attempt should be made to use the liquid of one manufacturer with the powder of another. Such an interchange would lead to unpredictable results. The dropper or the dropper bottle or squeeze bottle should be held vertically inverted while dispensing the liquid. It should be held away from the slab so that the drop does not touch the slab before it is released from the bottle. This rule holds good while dispensing any of the cement.

A slight excess of powder should be placed to one side on the mixing slab in the event it is needed to avoid re dispensing from the stock bottle during the mixing procedure. Solubility and strength are markedly altered by the powder - liquid ratio . The higher the ratio the better the properties. A typical powder - liquid ratio is 2.6 gms of powder to 1.0 ml of liquid for a primary consistency of cement.

Mixing slab:

A cool mixing slab should be employed . The temperature of the slab should not be below the dew point of the room lest moisture condenses on the surface and dilutes the cement. A temperature of 18deg. to 24deg. centigrade is indicated when room humidity permits. The moisture condensation upon a slab cooled down below the dew point, contaminates the mix ,diluting the liquid and shortening the setting time. Most chemical reactions are accelerated by the presence of heat because of an increase in molecular activity of the reactants. Since the combination of the zinc oxide and phosphoric acid results in liberation of heat in the immediate environment of reaction, this heat must be dissipated readily or the reaction will proceed too fast towards completion. Then ample working time is not available for proper manipulation of this cement. This is done by mixing the cement in a large surface area and by using a thick glass slab. A pre cooled glass slab also helps in achieving this.

Care of the liquid:

The liquid when exposed to humid atmosphere will absorb water whereas on exposure to dry air it will lose water. The cap should be replaced immediately after dispensing the liquid. The liquid is dispensed only after the powder is dispensed and just before the start of mixing. The material dispensed in syringes enables the mixed material to be syringed into place following mechanical mixing for 5 to 10 seconds.

Mixing:

The powder and liquid are preferably dispensed in a cool glass slab. A long narrow bladed stainless steel spatula is used and the powder is divided into 6 to 8 increments of smaller and larger sizes. Initially smaller increments are added one at a time and thoroughly spatulated in a large area of the slab to a creamy consistency. The initial smaller increments assist in neutralising the acid and reducing the large otherwise explosive exothermic reaction.. Then the larger increments are added with brisk rotary motion of the spatula to further saturate the liquid with newly forming complex zinc phosphates. Each increment may be spatulated for about 15 seconds. Incorporating smaller increments in the third part prevents the mix going beyond the desired ultimate consistency of the cement. Thus the mixing procedure begins and ends with small increments. The homogenity of the mass is attained by incorporating all the powder of each increment into the liquid and developing smoothness before the next powder portion is brought to the mixing area. 60 to 90 seconds of mixing appears to be an adequate length of time to accomplish a proper zinc phosphate cementing mass. The working time for this cement is about 3 to 6minutes. The setting time is about 5 to 14 minutes. Both these depend on the mixing procedure adopted.

Factors affecting setting and working time are:

1. Mixing over a large area extends working and setting time.

2. Rapid mixing shortens working and setting time.

3. Cooled glass slab extends working and setting time

4. Combination of cooled glass slab and incremental process ensures an adequate working time is maintained.

Setting time can be extended by a process known as slaking the fluid. Slaking is the process of adding small quantity of powder into the liquid about a minute before starting the main mixing procedure.

Properties:

Strength

The strength of ZPC is influenced by the initial composition of the powder and the liquid, P/L ratio, and the manner of mixing and the handling of the cement during its placement. ZPC has the ultimate compressive strength of all the materials which is about 14000-17000psi. It reaches the 2/3 the final strength in 1 hour.

The Tensile Strength is 3.1 to 4.5 psi
Elastic modulus is 9.3 to 13.4 psi

Before the reaction terminates and set has occurred, the contact of water with the cement tends to dilute the partially reacted liquid and leach out portions of cement. This weakens the cement and leaves a soft friable chalky surface. Proper isolation of the working area is therefore necessary until hardening has occurred.

Consistency and Film Thickness

Zinc phosphate cement can produce the lowest film thickness of all the cementing materials that is about 8 to 10μm. The final consistency should be fluid yet it will string up from the slab on the spatula about 2 to 3cm as the spatula is lifted away from the mass.

Dimensional Stability

ZPC exhibits a small, but negligible amount of shrinkage on hardening. The cement is porous and absorbs fluids resulting in dimensional increase.

Solubility and Disintegration

The cement is highly soluble in water for the first 24 hours after setting. And the loss of material can range from 0.04 to 3.3%. An acceptable upper limit is 0.2% by weight. After this time the solubility is much reduced. After the cement sets it is only slightly soluble in water but is still susceptible to acid attack in the presence of lactic acid. Increasing the water content of the liquid increases the solubility of the cement.

Biological Property:

ZPC is the most irritating of all the cements. The irritants are the acidity of the cement, microleakage, and the heat of the exothermic reaction.

Cementation:

The cement is added to the fitting surface and the casting seated before the cement matrix formation. After this it should be held under pressure until the cement sets in order to minimize air spaces. The patient may experience some pain during the cementation procedure. This is the result of both the low pH of the cement and the osmotic pressure caused by the movement of the fluid through the dentinal tubes. This will subside in a few hours.

Advantages of zinc phospate cement:

1. Easy to mix.
2. Has a sharp well defined set
3. Has sufficiently high compressive strength to resist forces of amalgam condensation.

Disadvantages of zinc phospate cement:

1. Has potential for pulpal irritation
2. No antibacterial action
3. Very brittle
4. No adhesive qualities
5. Susceptible to acid attack

ANHYDROUS ZINC PHOSPHATE CEMENTS/ HYDROPHOSPHATE CEMENTS.

An innovation in the compounding of ZPC is the mixing of dehydrated di-hydrogen phosphate of zinc, calcium and other metals, as well as the oxides of these metals with water. These so called water settable cements have been proposed to the same uses of luting and basing as the regular ZPC.

The mechanical properties of a hydrophosphate cement have been shown to be somewhat inferior to the acceptable values for compressive strength , film thickness, solubility and disintegration.

Acidity is similar to that of ZPC

This has no inherent superiority or clinical advantage over conventional ZPC

Partial hydration of the powder tends to occur resulting in variations of its characteristics.

COPPER PHOSPHATE CEMENT.

Copper or silver salts are sometimes used to replace portions of zinc oxides. This was basically done to provide a bactericidal property to the cement. Copper oxide added cement were found to give excellent retention of restorations to tooth when used as luting agent. These cements may be white, black or red colored depending on the type of oxide added to the powder. These are closely related to ZPC. It is supplied as powder and liquid.

Composition:

Powder

ZnO and copperoxide.

Liquid:

Aqueous solution of phosphoric acid.

Properties:

The two properties which distinguish this product from simple ZPC material is their black appearance and the bacericidal effect. Most properties are similar to conventional zinc phosphate cements but inferior to it.

Types:

Copper cements have been classified according to the percentage of copperoxide that is used as a replacement for ZnO.

Cupric oxide - Black

Cuprous oxide - red.

These cements are more acidic than phosphate cements. Strength is slightly higher. It is 21,000psi.

Manipulation:

Chemistry of the Cu elements is very similar to that of ZPC and they should be manipulated in the same manner.

Biological Property:

It has poor biological characteristics. It is highly irritant to the pulp tissue due to its very low pH. The pH of the cement may remain as low as 0.8 for many minutes.

GLASS IONOMER CEMENT

This cement was introduced by Wilson and Kent of England in 1972. This was a development to substitute the silicate cement which was a severe pulp irritant. The powder is basically silicate cement powder and the liquid is poly acrylic acid.

Presentation:

Type A: Pigmented Opalescent powder with clear viscous liquid

Type B: Pigmented Opalescent powder coated or added copolymer of polyacrylic acid.

Some common brands are, 'Ketac-Cem', 'Fuji Ionomer', and 'Chem-Bond', 'Aquacem'.

Composition:

Powder:

Silica	41.9
Alumina	28.6
Aluminium Fluoride	1.6
Calcium Fluoride	15.7
Sodium Fluoride	9.3
Aluminium Phosphate	3.8

Lanthium, strontium, and barium are added to provide radio opacity.

The fluorides serve as flux during the sintering process as well as provide anticariogenic property to this cement.

Liquid:

The liquid is primarily 50% Polyacrylic acid. It is copolymerised with itaconic acid, maleic acid, and tricarballic acid to adjust the viscosity. Tartaric acid is also a constituent and this is added to improve the workability of the cement. Addition of tartaric acid increases the working time and decreases the setting time of the cement. Water forms the next major component after polyacrylic acid.

Chemistry of Setting

The Glass Ionomer cement is formed by the reaction of three materials. A Fluoro alumino silicate glass powder and an ionic polymer of poly acrylic acid and water. An acid - base reaction occurs between the glass powder and the ionic polymer. Water is essential because that is the medium through which ion transfer take place. While mixing the powder and liquid, the acid slowly degrades the outer layer of glass particles, calcium ions and aluminium ions. During the early stages of setting, calcium ions are released more rapidly and is primarily responsible for reacting with the poly acid to form a reaction product that is calcium polysalts. Aluminium ions are released more slowly and become involved in setting at a later stage, often referred to as secondary reaction stage. The set material consists of unreacted glass cores embedded in a matrix of cross linked polyacid. The second stage of setting reaction involves the incorporation of significant quantities of aluminium in the matrix structure resulting in a marked maturation of the physical properties of the material. This stage requires about 24 hours and occurs when a polysalt matrix completely surrounds all of the initial reaction products. Although it may appear to be hard and set after the first 5 minutes, it truly takes a full day (24hours) before the material is completely set.

Mechanism of Adhesion:

The exact mechanism of adhesion of GIC to tooth structure is not well understood. It primarily involves the chelation of the carboxyl group of the poly salt to the calcium ions of the tooth structure. The bond strength to enamel is always higher than that to dentin.

Manipulation:

A prepared tooth surface should be cleaned with a slurry of pumice rinsed and then dried, but not dehydrated. Undue dessication opens up the tubules again enhancing penetration of the acidic liquid.

Proportioning:

P/L ratio varies 1.25 to 1.5 Gm powder to 1ml of liquid. The manufacturer given scoop and recommended number of drops of liquid from the dropper bottle are to be dispensed carefully on to the paper pad.

Mixing:

The powder and liquid are generally dispensed in a coated paper pad. The powder is introduced into the liquid in large increments and spatulated rapidly for 30 to 45 seconds. The properties of a Type I GIC are markedly influenced by manipulative factors. The cement is particularly susceptible to attack by water during setting . Therefore the accessible margins of the restoration have to be protected with varnish from attack by moisture.

Physical Properties:

General Properties:

Powder is finely ground with a particle size of 15µm. or less. The water settable systems tend to have somewhat longer working time. It is less stiff and more vulnerable to elastic deformation. Solubility in water during the first 24 hours is high.

Settind time of the cement is about	7mins.
Film thickness is	24µm.
Compressive strength 24hours	86MPa
Diametral Tensile strength 24 hours	6.2MPa
Modulus of Elasticity	7.3 Gpa
Solubility and disintegration in water	1.2weight %

Biological Properties:

This cement bonds to tooth structure. It prevents infiltration of oral fluid at the cement tooth interface. It is less irritant to the pulp tissue. The molecular size of the acid being high, its permeability into the dentinal tubules is less. Post cementation sensititvity is more with water settable formulations. The pH after 2 minutes is 2.33 and in 24 hours it is 5.67 and slightly more in water settable formulations. This pH values are related to the thinner mixes used for cementation.

Regardless of the type of ionomer cement formulations, when post operative sensitivity does occur, it is likely that one or more condition may exist. These conditions include a preexisting pulpitis, deep cavity preparation and associated minimal dentin thickness. Precaution should be taken to protect the pulp when cementing restorations with glass ionomer cements in deep cavities. The smear layer on the surface of the cavity preparation is best not to be removed. All deep areas of the preparation should be protected by a thin layer of hard setting calcium hydroxide cement.

The advantageous biological property of this cement is the provision of resistance to caries by means of leachable fluorides.

POLYCARBOXYLATE CEMENT

This cement was developed by Dennis Smith in 1960 in an effort to circumvent the potential pulpal problems associated with the low pH and the bio - compatibility problem related to the mobility of the small acidic ions into the dentinal tubules of the traditional zinc phosphate cement.

Dispensing:

Generally supplied as	TYPE-A	Powder and a liquid or
	TYPE-B	Water settable Powder.

Some common brands are: -

TYPE-A - 'Poly F', 'Durelon', 'Ceramco', 'P.C.A.', 'HARVARD CC', 'Carboxylon'

TYPE-B - 'Aquaset', 'Poly F Plus', 'Tylok', 'Poly-C',

Composition:

The cement powder is essentially similar to the zinc phosphate cement and contains zinc oxide and magnesium oxide. Part of the magnesium oxide may be replaced by stannic oxide to reduce the reactivity and adjust the working time. It may also contain stannous fluoride, which is basically added to help in the sintering of the cement by acting as a flux. But this also helps increase the strength of the cement and also provide the anticariogenic fluoride protection. Some contain smaller quantities of alumina, stainless steel fibers and also silica and bismuth salts. The water settable cements contain 15% to 18% polyacrylic acid coated on the powder particles.

The cement liquid is 32% to 42% polyacrylic acid in water. It has a molecular weight of about 25,000 to 50,000. Varying the molecular weight of the polymer can control the viscosity of the cement. The pH of the acid is adjusted by addition of sodium hydroxide. Itaconic acid and tartaric acid are also added to increase the shelf life of the liquid and to increase the working time. Liquid should be kept in a stoppered bottle, as loss of water from the liquid will lower its pH and slow down the setting. Liquid that appears cloudy after water loss should be discarded.

Manipulation:

Proportioning:

Powder - liquid ratio required to produce a cement of suitable consistency vary among brands, but they are in general range of 1.5 parts of powder to 1 part of liquid by weight. Cement mixed with water has a powder - liquid ratio of 5:1.

Mixing:

The material should be mixed on a surface that will not absorb liquid. A glass slab may be better than treated paper pad, which is generally supplied by the manufacturers, as it can be cooled. A non-absorptive surface is preferable because it will keep the liquid available for reaction and facilitates spatulation. Liquid should not be dispensed before the time that the mix is to be made. This is because it loses water very rapidly resulting in a marked increase in its viscosity. There is significant increase in viscosity even if the liquid is left on the slab for just a minute or two. The cement should be mixed within 30 to 60 seconds with half of all the powder being incorporated at once to provide the maximum length of working time which is 4.5 - 6 minutes. The working time can be extended to 10 - 15 minutes by mixing on a glass slab chilled to 4°C. This technique does not compromise on the strength of the mixed cement. The mix should not be too thin as it affects the strength, has a lower pH and makes the set material more soluble. Although the mix appears to be much thicker than a similar mix of zinc phosphate cement, it will flow readily into thin film when placed under pressure. The cement should be used while the surface is still glossy. If webbing occurs i,e. there is a loss of luster and a dull stringy rubber consistency, it means that the setting reaction has already started and a satisfactory film thickness and proper wetting of the tooth surface by the cement will no longer be possible.

Setting Time

In order that the final finishing procedures associated with the restoration can occur, setting time should be limited to 9 minutes and most cement conforms to this standard. The cement forming mechanism is thought to be a reaction of zinc ions with the polymeric acid via the carboxyl groups. Zinc can also react with the carboxyl groups of the adjacent polyacrylic acid chains so that an ionically crosslinked structure is formed. So the hardened cement consists of zinc oxide particles dispersed in a structure less matrix of zinc polycarboxylate. Fresh mobile cement paste wets and adheres to the enamel apatite surface by hydrogen bonds provided by free carboxylic acid groups. As the cement reaction proceeds, most of these hydrogen bonds are replaced by metal ions to give metal ion bridges that provide adhesion of the cement to the enamel. There is some evidence that the cement may also bond to the collagen of the dentin. Collagen contains some branched chains that terminate in carboxylate acid groups and others that terminate in amino groups. The former can link to the cement mass by metal ion bridging, while the latter group bond by hydrogen bridges. Sodium fluoride does not enter the setting reaction but is released to the surrounding tooth structure. The matrix structure is amorphous and porous to some extent. During setting, heat is given out since the reaction is exothermic.

Setting time depends on :

(A) The powder - This is generally prepared commercially by heating the ingredients to above 1000°C , causing granulation, by a sintering process. Subsequently the solid is ground to a very fine powder. The rate of reaction of the powder with the liquid depends on:

1. The temperature, to which it is heated, a higher temperature reduces the reactivity of the powder.

2. The particle size after grinding to a finer material reacts more quickly, since a greater surface area is exposed to the liquid.

(B) Manipulative variable:

Four factors will accelerate the setting reaction

1. High powder-liquid ratio
2. Fast rate of addition of powder to liquid.
3. Presence of moisture.
4. Higher temperature.

(C) Tartaric acid added to control the setting reaction.

Properties:

Strength:

Compressive strength of this cement is inferior to ZPC. Compressive strength is around 7250psi. Studies have shown that cements of this strength or greater will retain castings satisfactorily with good fit. 24-hour compressive strength of poly acrylate cement for luting is 8300 - 14400psi, which is much lower than that of zinc phosphate cement which has a value of 14,000- 19,000psi. However the tensile strength of polyacrylate cement is about 40% higher than zinc phosphate cement. Modulus of elasticity is about 1/3 that of zinc phosphate cement mixed for a luting consistency. Strength of polycarboxylate cement appears to be less sensitive than ZPC to small fluctuation in P/L ratio. Reducing the recommended amount of powder in the mix of polycarboxylate cement by 1/3 reduces the strength by 5MPa(700psi) or about 9%. On the other hand a comparable reduction in the amount of powder incorporated into a mix of ZPC reduces the strength by about 35% as compared with that attained with the recommended ratio.

Film Thickness

Although polycarboxylate mix prepared with correct powder liquid ratio and proper manipulation appears to be very thick and viscous, as compared with corresponding mixes of ZPC, it will form a film of 25µm or less. It meets the requirement that has been established for the cementation of precision fillings and castings. The viscous appearance of the cement is misleading in that it is no more difficult to seat a precise fitting casting with polycarboxylate than ZPC.

Bond Strength

An interesting feature of polycarboxylate cement is its bonding to enamel and dentin. Bond strength to enamel is about 3.45 to 13.1MN/m^2 (500 to 1900psi). Bond strength to dentin is about 300psi. Optimum bonding however requires clean tooth surface. Bonding of polyacrylate cement to gold casting alloy is likewise highly dependent of surface preparation. Sandblasting or electrolytic etching of the gold alloy surface is necessary to achieve optimum bonding. Failure usually occurs cohesively or at the cement-metal interface. The cement metal interface debonding is because the cement is unable to bond to the metal in the chemically dirty condition. So chemically dirty surface on the cavity side of the casting should be removed in order to provide a mechanical bond at cement - metal interface. The cement can be carefully abraded with a small stone or by using air borne abrasive. Also adhesive bonding can be attained by electroplating the casting with tin and thereby obtain a bond through the reaction of carboxyl group in the cement and the tin.

Solubility

Solubility in water at one day varies from 0.12% to 0.25%.

Dimensional Stability

It shows linear contraction when setting at 37°C. The amount of contraction varies from 1% for a wet specimen at 1 day to 6% for a dry specimen at 14 days.

Viscosity

Viscosity after a couple of minutes is less than that of ZPC even though the viscosity of PCC was initially higher. The freshly mixed PCC has the property of being pseudo plastic and show shear thinning on mixing. This means that although the material may appear to be too thick to flow properly while it is being placed, the pressure that is exerted makes it flow quite satisfactorily. Cement will reach 80% of its final strength within 1hour.

Biological Properties:

It is minimally irritating to the PD organ. Although the pH of the setting cement is in the range of 1.6 to 3.6 for the first day or so, it is minimally irritating because of the giant dimension of the polyacrylic acid macro molecules and their attachment to the main bulk of the cement mass. The acid has low diffusion mobility into the underlying dentin due to its immediate complexing with the dentinal fluoride, calcium and some proteinaceous components. The complex product will prevent further penetration of the acid. This will result in minimal effect on PD organ unless it comes in actual contact with the pulp tissue and moreover the dissociation of the acid is very weak.

The Effect At Different Effective Depths :

Whenever PD organ has 1mm effective depth or greater, a healthy reparative reaction can be expected.

Whenever the material comes in contact with the pulp a destructive reaction will definitely be initiated.

RESIN CEMENT

A plethora of resin based cements have now become available for luting. These were primarily developed to cement Maryland bridges and other non-preparation bridges and splints. This increase is due to improved properties of filled resins over the years and the advent of dentin bonding agents. Resin cements are now available for specific uses such as attachment of orthodontic brackets, resin-bonded bridges and for luting all ceramic inlays and onlays. Availability of dual cure resins cements has led to better bio-compatiblty of the material.

Presentation:

Polymer, monomer and catalysts are the important constituents. They may be supplied in two system packs or more number, in which case they are all independently packed. The common presentations are:

Powder and liquid, laste and liquid, liquid and liquid, or paste and paste system when in two component packs or powder, liquid or paste, forming any of the three important components of the resin system.

Some common brands available are 'Sevriton', ' Super Bond C & B', 'Comspan', 'Conclude', 'Panavia Ex', 'Scotchbond Resin Cement', 'Opal Luting Composite'.

The 4-meta resin cements claim mechanical bonding to enamel and chemical bonding to both oxidized precious and base metal alloys. E.g.: 'Super Bond C&B'.

Composition:

It is similar to that of many modern resin based composite filling materials. This also contains an organic matrix and a silane treated fillers. The resin matrix is usually BISGMA or UDMA, also incorporates monomers with functional groups that have been used to induce bonding to dentin, because most of the prepared tooth surface is dentin. They include Organo phosphonates, Hydroxy ethyl metharylate (HEMA) and 4-methacryl-ethyl tri mellitic anhydride (4-META) system. Bonding of cements to enamel can be obtained through the acid etch technique. Polymerization can be achieved by the conventional peroxide-amine induction system or by light activation. Several systems use both mechanisms and are referred to as dual cure - which are most acceptable to ensure complete polymerization of all deeper aspect of the restorations.

Fillers used in resin cements are finer in size to ensure thinner film thickness. Best preferred filler would be 70% by volume. Hybrid filler particle made of soft barium or strontium rather than quartz. Soft small particle fillers are widely used in resin cements.

Manipulation:

The two component systems are generally mixed in a coated paper pad to initiate the polymerization. The mixing time is usually 20 - 30 seconds. This often incorporates air, which lowers wear resistance. Light cured systems are single component systems, which are activated by light energy. Time of exposure to light should be for a period of minimum of 30 seconds. They are widely used for cementation of porcelain and glass ceramic restorations and for direct bonding of ceramic orthodontic brackets and in case of porcelain restoration is done in the center with 14mm diameter tip. Each lateral surface is cured for 10 seconds. Distance of curing tip from resin should be less than 1 mm, if that is not possible the curing time should be increased. Angle of contact is preferably 90°. The dual cure cements are two component systems. They require mixing that is similar to the chemically activated system. The chemical activation is slow and provides extended working time until the cement is exposed to the curing light at which point the cement solidifies rapidly. It then continues to gain strength over an extended period because of chemically activated polymerization.

The time of excess removal is critical. It is important to apply a separating medium to adjacent soft tissues and teeth in the absence of rubberdam.

Properties:

Resin based cements are often designed for specific applications rather than general uses. They are formulated to provide the handling characteristic required for the particular application. E.g. Cements recommended for cementation of indirect restoration have film thickness of 25 μm or less. Cement that is indicated for direct bonding of orthodontic brackets would not have the same handling characteristics or properties desired for a crown or bridge cement.

With respect to bonding to dentin the so-called adhesive cements which incorporate the phosphonates, HEMA, 4-META adhesion system generally develop reasonably good bond strength to dentin. Some commercial resin based cements furnish a bonding agent as a separate component of the cement system. Bonding to the tooth structure may be more critical for resin based cements than for some other types of cements, because they posses no anticariogenic potential.

Biological Properties:

Resin cements just like the composite restorative resins are irritating to the pulp. Uncured resin increases the pulpal irritation and to prevent this dual cure material are used. Pulp protection via a calcium hydroxide or glass ionomer liner is important in deeper preparation. Dentin bonding system does help in sealing the dentin and preventing pulpal irritation.

NEWER LUTING CEMENTS

These are a new class of cements. They are glass ionomer cements modified with resin compositions. They have the benefits of both the conventional glass ionomer cements and the composite resins. It is supposed to have the chemical adhesion to the tooth structure and the fluoride protection to tooth similar to that imparted by the conventional glass ionomer cements and as well as the esthetics, micro mechanical retention to the enamel and dentin of tooth and to prepared metal surface of retorations. They also have a chemical bonding to the etched, silanated surface of ceramic restorations. With these properties these cements would be the ideal choice for thin esthetic veneer restorations.

Some of the common brands are:

'Dyract Cem', 'Fuji Duet', 'Vitremer Luting Cement'

Presentation:

This is usually supplied as powder and liquid. Different surface conditioning or treatment agents are available to be used on the bonding tooth and restoration surfaces.

Setting Reaction:

It sets chemically by an acid base reaction similar to glass ionomer cement, by photo polymerization similar to a resin cement and sometime a third mechanism of reduction-oxidation also helps the organic portion of the cement to harden. It is hence a dual cure cement or a triple cure hardening cement.

Manipulation:

Powder and liquid are dispensed according to the manufacturers instructions using the scoop and dropper bottle provided. The cement powder is incorporated into the liquid in two increments and spatulated thoroughly into a creamy paste. It has extended working time. In total darkness the cement usually takes about 15 minutes or more to set hard. On exposure to photocuring light the surface immediately hardens and protects the moisture critical chemically setting components within the cement. So this does not require surface protection using varnish. The cement has to be exposed to light for 30 to 60 seconds.

Properties:

All mechanical properties fall intermediate between glass ionomer cement and resin cement. The key advantages of this cement are its :

Excellent long lasting esthetic property,

Fluoride leaching and hence anticaries,

Very low solubility in oral fluids as well as acids in the oral cavity,

Bonding to dentin and elimination of microleakage.

Resistance to staining,

Durable margins,

Low film thickness (15μm).

Radio-opacity

THE CHOICE OF LUTING CEMENT

All the available luting cements are capable of working successfully. The choice of which to use in a given case will depend upon the presenting clinical circumstance. The choice of cement is mandated to a large extent by the functional and biologic requirement of the clinical situation. The factors that determine the choice of the cement for luting are the :

Proximity of the pulp

Age of the patient

Need for additional retention

Caries incidence of the patient

Ease of handling

Chemical properties of the cement with relation to the tooth and the restoration

Physical properties of the cements with relation to the function of the tooth and restoration.

Esthetic requirement.

REFERENCES

1. FX1000P1. Skinner's- Science of Dental Materials
   - Ralph W. Phillips, 8th Edi-W.B. Saunders 1982
2. Phillips - Science of Dental Materials
   - Kenneth J. Anusavice,10th Edi- W.B. Saunders1996.
3. Operative Dentistry - Modern Theory and Practice
   - M.A. Marzouk, 1st Edi-All India Publishers, 1997.
4. The Art and Science of Operative Dentistry
   - Clifford M. Sturdevant, 3rd Edi-Mosby-Year Book, 1995.
5. Restorative Dental Materials - Robert G. Craig, 8th Edi
   -C.V. Mosby, 1989.
6. Recent Advances in Operative Dentistry A. Parameswaran and K.S.Karthikeyan - FODI,1985
7. Text Book of Operative Dentistry - Lloyd Baum - 3rd Edi
   - W.B.Saunders,1995
8. Pickard's Manual of Operative Dentistry E.A.M.Kidd and B.G.N. Smith,6th Edi - ELBS,1992
9. Operative Dental Surgery - J.J.Messing and G.E.Ray, 2nd Edi The Macmillan Press, 1982
10. Materials used in dentistry lecture series the Tamilnadu Dr.M.G.R Medical University, 1996.
11. Notes on Dental Materials - E.C.Combe,5th Edi Churchill Livingston,1986
12. Dr.S.Balagopal - Tensile Bond Strength of three Dentine Adhesives - 1987.

CRUISE FOR GAMMA 2 FREE AMALGAM.

Jagannathan K.

Dental amalgam is one of the dental biomaterial in the spectrum of direct posterior long term restorative materials. It serves as the benchmark to compare the wear properties of newer restorative materials. This is the only self sealing material, wears as natural tooth. It serves as long term restoration, in indicated cases when well manipulated.

Indicated in posterior class 1, class 2, endodontic access sealing in posterior teeth, core build ups in posterior endodontically treated teeth with appropriate lining including dentine bonding agents.

Its use in root end filling debated in the recent years. At the present time not used in class 5; access seal in the anterior endodonticaly treated teeth; or as die material.

Non tooth color; galvanism; thermal conductivity; discoloration; tarnish; corrosion; allergic for very few people; potential toxicity due to mercury; poor tensile strengths are negative areas

Adequate compressive strength; self sealing when there is minimal surface corrosion; long track records are the positive areas.

THE GRAY AREAS ARE VARIABILITY IN MANIPULATION.

Successful amalgam restoration depends on multiple factors. One of the factor is trituration. Even though recent western dental biomaterial text strongly recommends high speed amalgamator for triturating modern amalgam alloys, hand (mortar - pestle) trituration continued in developing country..

The essential difference between traditional and modern dental amalgam alloys is the elimination of gamma 2 phase and to obtain eta phase in the set amalgam microstructure

Research and development in dental amalgam have shown a reverse stand in the dimensional changes. Historically, we expected a slight setting expansion and at the present time we expect a slight net contraction. Modern amalgam alloy shows net contraction when triturated with minimal mercury in a high speed amalgamator. Well proportioned modern dental amalgam alloy and mercury, when triturated in a high speed amalgamator yields an amalgam that contains optimal amount of reacted and unreacted phases and virtual elimination of gamma 2 phase.

Dental amalgam alloys require more mercury when hand triturated in mortar ano pestle. Hand trituration produces more gamma 1, less than optimal gamma, mercury rich eta and gamma 2 even in high copper amalgam alloy.

The purpose of the presentation is to emphasize high speed amalgamator for modern amalgam alloys and strong recommendation of not teaching and practicing hand trituration.

The dispensing spectrum to be reduced to pre dosed single use capsules alone. High speed amalgamator alone should be used.Smaller lathe cut or spherical particles are needed depending on the contour restorations

Pathway towards better dental amalgamation.

Modern amalgam alloy	*Traditional amalgam alloy*
Has a potential to eliminate gamma 2 phase if optimal mercury: alloy ratio is used in high speed amalgamator	Has no potential to eliminate gamma 2 phase
Can form gamma 2 phase when triturated by hand since mercury: alloy ratio is not optimal	Always form gamma 2 phase
Eta phase formed in lieu of gamma 2	Not appericible amount of eta formed

Mercury rich eta phase will be formed when hand triturated.

More gamma 1 will form and lead to setting expansion

Less unreacted gamma leads to poor strength

Presence of gamma 2 leads to mercuroscopic expansion

Mercury rich eta phase leads to corrosion more than with optimal eta phase containing amalgam

HIGH COPPER AMALGAM ALLOY WILL YIELD AN AMALGAM OF LOW COPPER TYPE.

The aim of this presentation is to highlight the prophetic statement "The more mercury that is mixed with alloy, the greater will be the amount retained in the amalgam" by Phillips R.W. & Boyd D.A., (1947) and foresight of minimal mercury technique by Eames (1959).

The presentation is aimed at optimal manipulation of the dental amalgam in order to have a ideal restorative material which will have the expected properties with due respect to Mercury hygiene.

Amalgamation is by optimal dissolution and crystallization. Low Mercury : Alloy ratio favours best possible amalgam. The amount of unreacted alloy Gamma phase favours strength proper amount of Gamma, Gamma 1 (AgHg) formation avoids expansion, reduces creep, improves overall properties of amalgam. Gamma 2 (SnHg) phase elimination and eta phase

(Copper Tin) is possible only low Mercury alloy ratio and this in turn possible with high speed amalgamators. Copper Tin eta phase also the weakest phase in corrosion resistance. Pure Copper Tin Crystals are strong and resistant to corrosion. But Copper tin crystal formed in the presence of Hg considered to be weak and less corrosion resistant.

Hence a technic conscious manipulation of amalgam and rigid protocol of mercury management can make dental amalgam as a useful restorative material.

REFERENCES

1. David Brown — Dental amalgam BDJ APR 23, 1988
2. Greener E.H. — Amalgam - Yesterday, Today and Tomorrow oper dent 4;24-35, 1979.
3. Maxwell H. Anderson — Dental Amalgam DCNA 37;3;419-431 JULY 1993.
4. Ogletree & Marek — Effect of Mercury on corrosion cu-sn eta phase in dental amalgams Dent Mater 11;323-336 SEP 1995.
5. Jagannathan K. — Amalgam, Amalgamation Amalgamator Materials used in Dentistry J.J. Kannappan

PROPERTIES OF DENTAL MATERIALS AND THEIR APPLICATIONS

Kandaswamy D.

INTRODUCTION :

The dental materials are usually developed by the producer and selected and utilised by the dentist. This requires a complete understanding of their properties and their application in dentistry. No single property can be used as a measure of quality for the materials. Hence it is imperative to know the mechanical, chemical and biological properties of the materials, the principles behind such properties and their application to a given situation.

The task of making a material perform is made more difficult by the dynamic environment in the oral cavity.

For eg. The occlusal load that acts on a restoration is high in magnitude, varying in direction and is intermittent in nature causing an impact, continuous or cyclic stresses.

This underlines the importance for a thorough understanding of the different properties and their application in the oral cavity.

PHYSICAL PROPERTIES

When a force acts on a body to produce a deformation, a resistance is developed to this external force which is called stress.

Stress :

It is the internal reaction to the external force. It is equal in intensity and opposite in direction to the external force. It is distributed over a given area of a body.

Stress = Force/Area

Forces in the Oral Cavity are of 3 types.

FORCES

- Continuous (Constantly Present)
- Impact (One time Force)
- Cyclic (Multiple Impacts)

The direction of force determines the type of stress.

FORCE
(TWO SETS OF FORCES)

- Acting in the same straight Line
  - Directed away From each other → Leads to Elongation → Tensile Stress
  - Directed Towards Each other → Compression (or) Shortening → Compressive Stress
- Acting Parallel to Each Other → Twisting or Sliding → Shear Stress

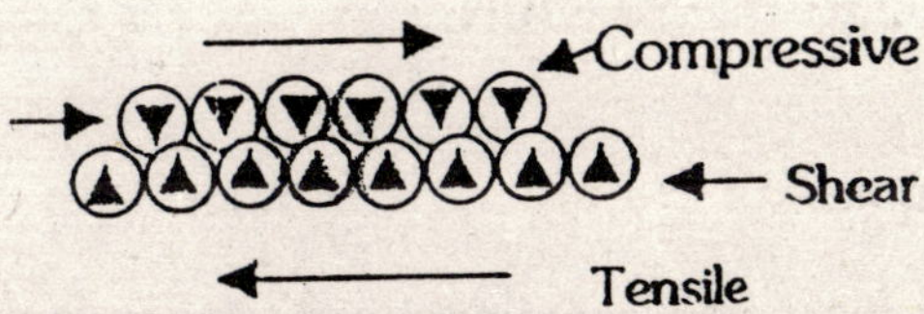

Each type of stress is capable of producing a corresponding deformation in the body.

Strain :

It is a change in length occuring per unit length of the material due to stress.

$$\text{Strain} = \frac{\text{Change in Length}}{\text{Original Length}}$$

Complete understanding of these two phenomena is essential to study the different propeties.

Stress Strain Curve :

If the measurement of the load and the resultant deformation is plotted in a graph after converting them to Stress and Strain the following graph will result

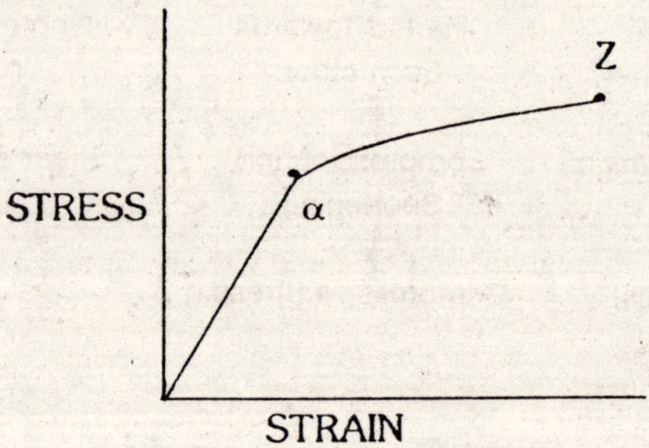

A typical curve shows a linear or straight line upto a point α after which it is concave towards the strain axis.

The curve ends at pt Z where fracture occurs.

The linear portion of the curve denotes the proportionality of stress to strain upto the point α

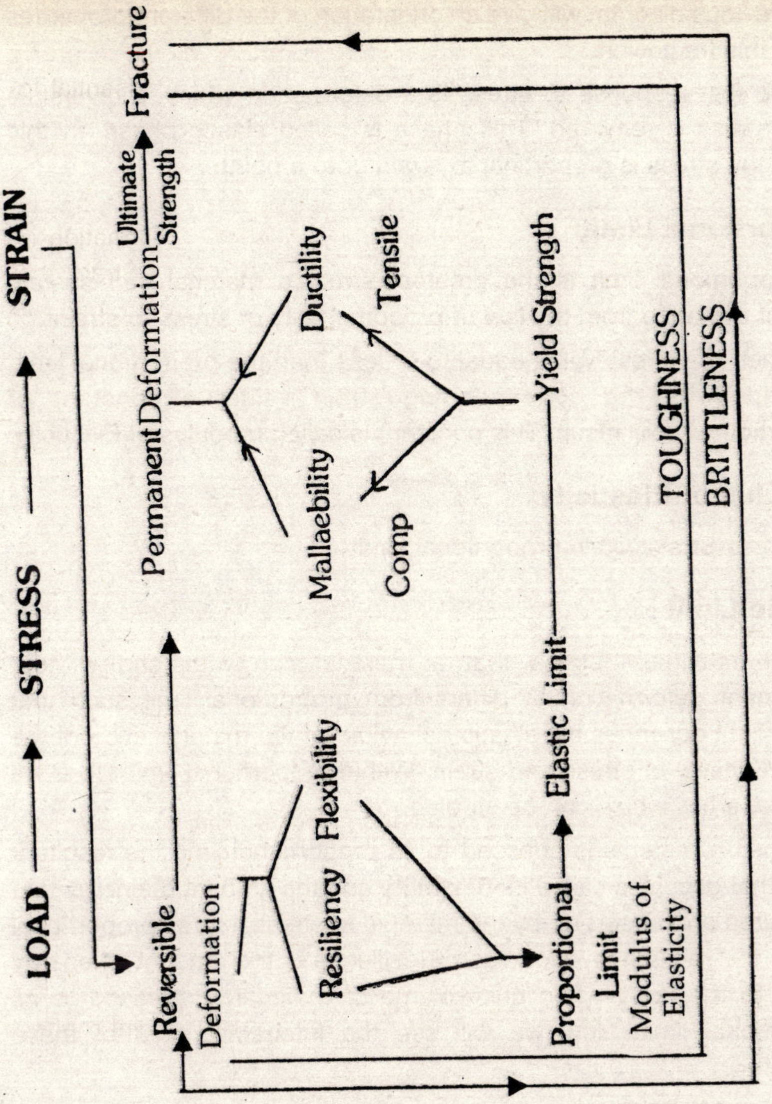
LOAD
STRESS
STRAIN
Reversible Deformation
Permanent Deformation
Ultimate Strength
Fracture
Resiliency
Flexibility
Mallaebility
Ductility
Comp
Tensile
Proportional Limit
Modulus of Elasticity
Elastic Limit
Yield Strength
TOUGHNESS
BRITTLENESS

Force or load causing stress resulting in strain has been described. The previous diagram will give an orientation of the different properties within this framework.

The first response to stress is a deformation which is reversible when stress is removed. This phase is called elastic phase. In this phase the stress is proportinal to strain upto a point.

Proportional Limit:

Proportional limit is the greatest strain a material can sustain without deviating from the law of proportionality of stress to strain.

When the stress value equal to or less than the proportional limit, is divided by the corresponding strain value, a constant of proportionality will result. This constant is called modulus of Elasticity.

Modulus of Elasticity:

Stress/Strain within proportional Limit

Elastic Limit :

The maximum stress that a material can withstand without permanent deformation. It differs from proportional limit such that elastic limit describes the elastic behaviour of the material and not the proportionality of stress and strain. Within proportional limit there are two properties which can be studied.

When a material is stressed to its proportional limit the resultant strain that occurs is called its **flexibility** and the amount of energy that is required and absorbed by the material to stress it to its proportional limit is the **resilience.** Modulus of resilience is the amount of energy stored in the body when unit volume of material is stressed to its proportional limit. Now we will see the interrelationship of these properties.

$$\text{Modulus of Elasticity} = \frac{\text{Proportional Limit}}{\text{Maximal Flexibility}}$$

Beyond the elastic limit the material begins to enter the plastic stage in which the permanent deformation occurs.

Yield Strength :

The stress at which a material begins to function in a plastic manner. At this stress, a limited amount of permanent deformation has occurred. This leads on to the plastic stage or the permanent deformation stage.

Permanent deformation occurs when a material is stressed beyond its elastic limit.

Stress ⟶ Elastic Limit ⟶ Permanent Deformation

PERMANENT DEFORMATION

↓

Tensile Stress → Ductility

Compressive Stress → Malleability

Ductility:

Ductility is the ability of the material to withstand permanent deformation under a tensile load without rupture.

Malleability:

Malleability is the ability to withstand permanent deformation under a compressive load without fracture. If the material is stressed beyond permanent deformation then fracture results.

The amount of energy required to stress the material to the point of fracture is the toughness of the material

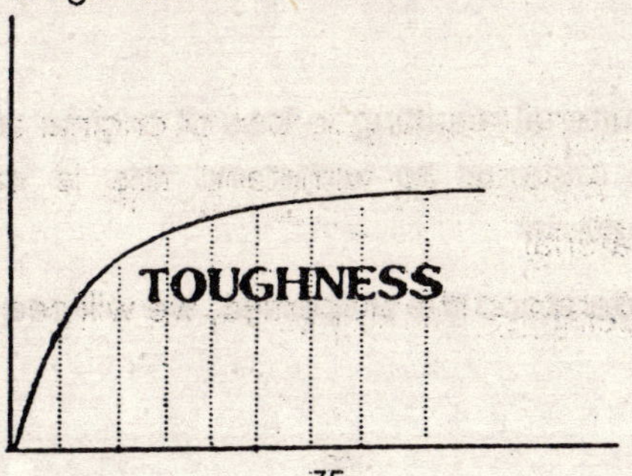

The maximum stress that is required to cause fracture is called ultimate strength

Strength : The maximal stress required to cause a fracture.

STRENGTH

- Tensile → Resistance to Tensile Stress
- Compressive → Resistance to Compressive Stress
- Shear → Resistance to Shear stress

STRENGTH

- Impact Strength → Energy required to fracture by a impact force
- Flexure Strength → Energy required to fracture under a static load
- Fatigue Strength → Repeated cyclic forces requried to cause a fracture below the ultimate strength

Impact Strength :

Impact strength is the ability to withstand impact forces. Impact strength is directly proportional to the resilience of the material and inversely proportional to the modulus of elasticity.

Hardness :

It is the ability of the material to withstand indentation.

Wear :

Is the loss of material resulting in loss of original anatomical form. The ability of the material to withstand this is called the wear resistance of the material

Now having understood the properties, we will see the importance of their application.

Normal Biting force

The biting forces vary from 390 N to 880 N from the first and second molars to 55 N at the incisors. In children from 6 - 17 Years of age there is an increase of 22.2 N for every year. The factors that act on the chewing side and opposite side are almost similar. There is a difference in the biting force between men and women (in Women it is less by 89N). Forces acting on the fixed bridge partial dentures and complete dentures are much less than that in the normal dentition. The maximum force measured on the partial denture or complete denture is 115N compared to 752N for natural dentition.

The physical properties of a restoration must be suitable to withstand stress applied by the repetitive forces of mastication. With a constant force, the stress is inversely proportional to the contact area. The stress can be reduced by :

1. Increasing the area over which the force is acting
2. By using materials with high strength properties
3. By Increasing the bulk of the material
4. By designing the restoration and appliances in such a way to avoid sharp line angles, non uniform areas, scratched, notched, or pitted surfaces.
5. The base materials under a restoration must have a high modulus of elasticity.
6. The material must have a high resilience to withstand the impact forces in the oral cavity.

The proportional limit, elastic limit and yield strength are important properties. There are certain conditions where the forces should not exceed these limits like a fixed bridge which will result in permanent deformation if the yield strength is exceeded.

Certain conditions require the material to have a permanent deformation eg. In constructing an orthodontic appliance.

It is necessary to introduce a stress in excess of yield strength to permanently bend them.

The ultimate strength decides the size or cross sectional area of the restoration.

Fatigue strength is an important factor in designing a restoration. Therefore it is important to know the amount of stress it can withstand for an essentially unlimited number. of cycles.

A material with a high value for elongation can be bent permanently without the danger of fracture.

Malleability:

Shows the ability of the metal to be rolled into sheets without fracture. Ductility is related to burnishing of a material on the margins of a casting.

Resilience:

Is important in evaluation of orthodontic wire since the amount of work expected from a particular spring in moving a tooth is of interest.

Since toughness is represented as a area, a material can be tough by having a combination of high proportional limit and ultimate strength and moderately high strain at rupture or by having a moderately high proportional limit and ultimate strength and a large strain at rupture.

ANALYSIS OF THE STRESS - STRAIN CURVE

The shape of the stress strain curve and the magnitude of the stress and strain will allow classification of material with respect to their properties.

For eg. The longitudinal portion of the curve is closer to the long axis, the material is stiff and not flexible.

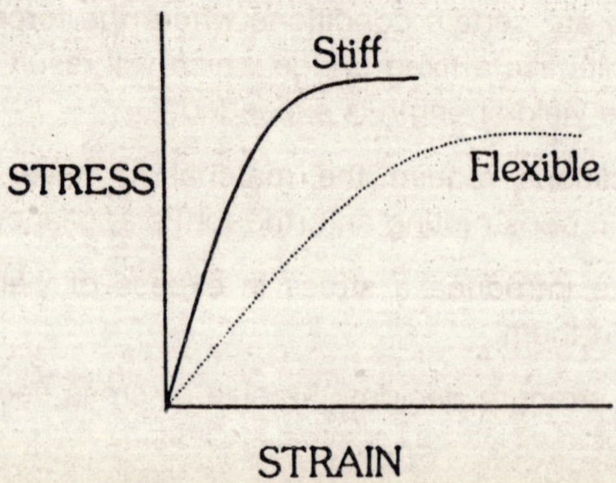

If it is away from the long axis the material is flexible

If the fracture occurs after a long concave portion of the curve it denotes that the material is tough and ductile.

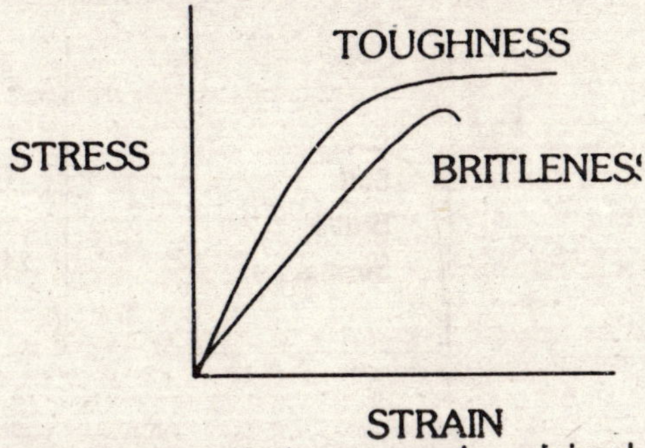

If the elastic portion of the curve is minimal, it denotes the brittleness of the material.

If the longitudinal portion of the curve is longer, then the material is strong.

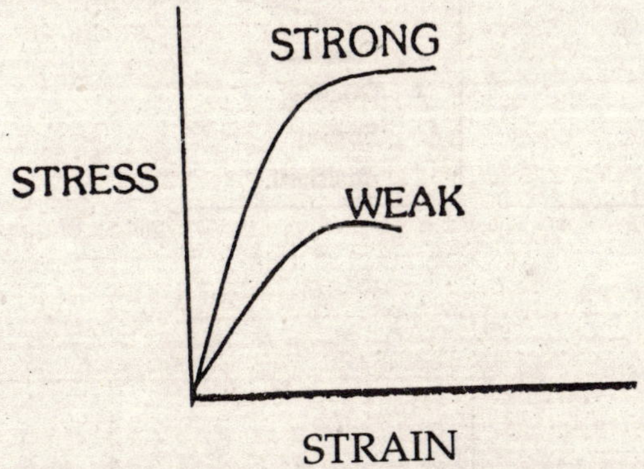

If the longitudinal portion is short, then the material is weak.

Hence from a stress-strain curve, it is possible to have a combination of properties and select the required material

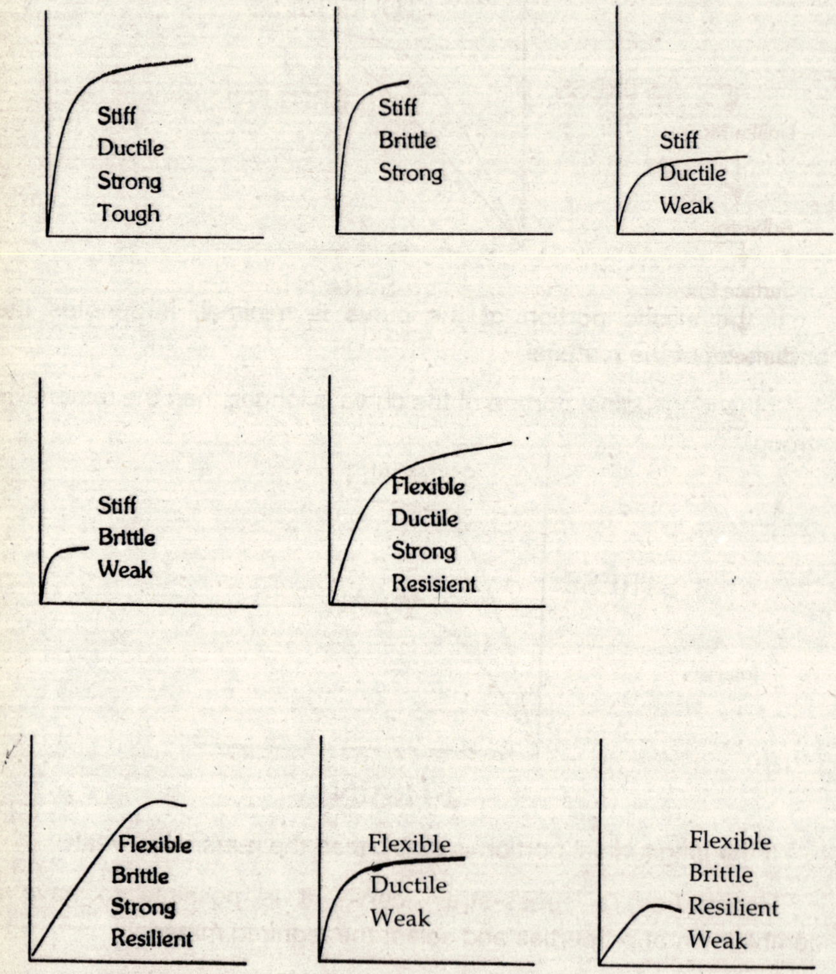

Stiff
Ductile
Strong
Tough
Stiff
Brittle
Strong
Stiff
Ductile
Weak
Stiff
Brittle
Weak
Flexible
Ductile
Strong
Resisient
Flexible
Brittle
Strong
Resilient
Flexible
Ductile
Weak
Flexible
Brittle
Resilient
Weak

Now we will discuss the attraction between different materials and the properties which determine them.

ATTRACTION BETWEEN SUBSTANCES

- Attraction of molecules (Chemical Bonding)
  - Unlike Molecules → Adhesion
  - Same Kind of Molecules → Cohesion
  - Adhesion / Cohesion → Surface Energy → Surface Tension → Capillarity
  - Adhesion / Cohesion → Wettability → Contact Angle
- Mechanical Bonding → Microscopic and Sub Microscopic Retention

SOLIDS

- Energy in the Interior → Atoms are Equally Attracted. Interatomic distance is equal to the energy in the molecule
- Energy at the surface → Outer most atoms are not equally attracted in all the directions. Energy is more → Surface Energy, Surface Tension

SURFACE ENERGY

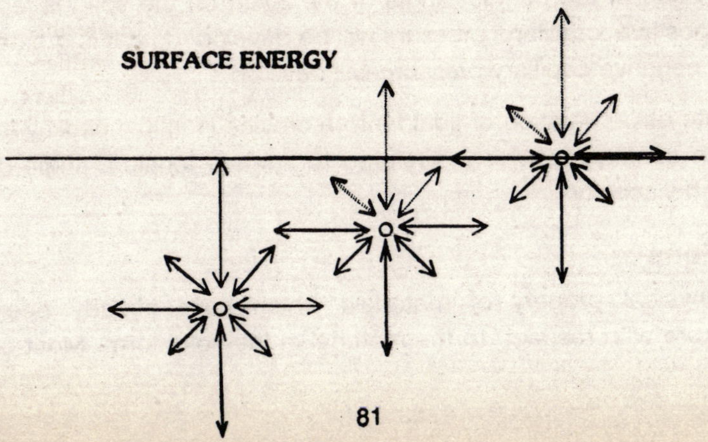

Bonding between surface atoms of two material to minimise the surface energy is called - Adhesion

The roughness on the surface of any materials will not allow adhesion of the total surface area. Only the hills or high spots on the surface of two materials will come into contact.

This can be overcome by allowing a fluid to flow into these irregularities and increase the contact area. This is called wetting.

Wetting depends on

Cleanliness of the surface | Surface energy

The angle formed by the adhesive or wetting agent over the adherend determine the wetting ability. This angle is called the contact angle.

Smaller the contact angle, better the wettability

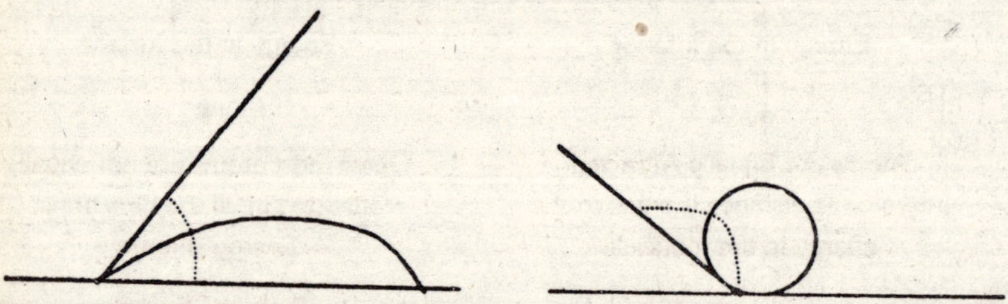

The penetration of liquids into narrow crevices is known as capillary action. If the contact angle of the liquid on the solid is less than 90°, positive capillary pressure will be developed . It if is greater than 90°, negative capillary pressure will develop.

The rate of penetration of liquid into a crevice is influenced by its penetration coefficient, which is related to surface tension, angle of contact and viscosity.

Applications :

The physical propery of materials which have already been discussed are with respect to the material in the solid form. Most of the materials used in dentistry are in liquid state during some stage of fabrication. Certain materials are amorphous like waxes or resins which exhibit properties of liquid when under stress. Some materials are also used as liquids.

So a complete understanding of the properties is essential for their application in dentistry. Restorative dentistry depends on relationship between restoration and tooth substance. Best results are achieved when these two substances are brought together in the best possible manner. The relationship between those two subtances is dictated by surface energy of materials to begin with. We have already discussed how the surface energy or surface tension can be lowered by use of surfactant.

A classical example of reducing surface tension to increase wettability is the use of a surfactant on wax when hand investing technique is used.

By reducing surfacing tension, increased wettability is brought about, by the decrease in contact angle of the liquid.

For water the contact angle with wax is high.

The spreading of water on wax when a surfactant is added is the result of decreased contact angle.

Molecules of water	Surfactant
↕ Cohesive forces	Molecules inserted between water molecules
↕ Surface Tension	↓ Cohesive forces between water molecules
Does not wet the surface of wax	→ Better wettability

One more example of wetting of surfaces by liquids include the spreading of molten flux on hot metal during melting on soldering operation.

Trituration of amalgam is also an example of the mercury wetting the alloy particles.

Contact angle is determined not only by the surface tension of the liquid, it varies with the material with which it is used. Therefore it is imperitive to select the suitable liquid for each material.

Example : Water with glass 14°

Water with Acrylic 75°

It also varies with Temperature Viscosity, Flow, Penetration Coefficient, Capillarity of liquid. All these properties play a important role in bonding agents.

THERMAL PROPERTIES

The properties of the same material varies with variations in temperature

The thermal properties of a dental material must be studied because

1) The Intra oral temperature is higher than the temperature outside.

2) Variation of temperature occur inside the oral cavity.

The thermal properties of a material placed inside the oral cavity must be compatible with that of the oral tissues, namely tooth structure and the oral soft tissues. So a complete understanding of these properties is required.

Thermal properties of a material arise either due to conduction of heat through the material, or due to absorption of heat by the material.

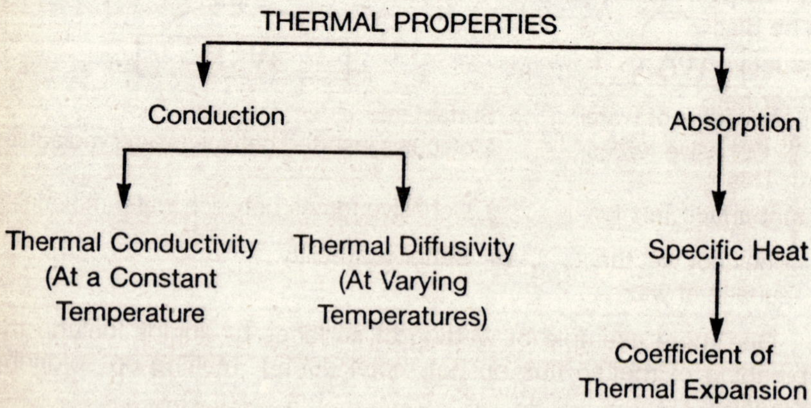

Thermal conductivity:

Thermal conductivity of the material is the quantity of heat that passes through a unit mass of the material in one second, when the thermal gradient across the material is 1°C. However, such a constant thermal gradient is seldom possible in the oral cavity, because within the mouth the thermal gradient varies constantly. . In such situation thermal diffusivity is used to assess the transient heat conducted through the material at a particular temperature. It is given by the formula :

$$\text{Thermal Diffusivity} = \frac{\text{Thermal Conductivity}}{\text{Specific Heat X Density}}$$

Specific heat of a material is the quantity of heat required to raise the temperature of unit mass of the substance by 10C.

The effect of heat absorption by a material is a change in its dimension. When measured in one dimension, it is called **coefficient of linear expansion,** which is the change in length per unit length of the material, when the temperature is raised or lowered by 1°C.

Application:

The application of thermal properties requires a knowledge of the thermal properties of enamel and dentin. For instance, the thermal conductivity of a material determines how much heat is going to be conducted from the restoration to the tooth.

INSULATING PROPERTY OF MATERIALS

A material with poor thermal conductivity is a good insulator, and can be placed beneath a metallic restoration which has a high thermal conductivity. The combination of an insulator and a conductor in this manner help the dentist to achieve good results.

At the same time, denture base materials are poor conductors of heat. This prevents the adequate exchange of heat between the denture base and the oral tissues, thus causing discomfort to the patient. The patient is unable to precieve the correct temperatures in his/her mouth.

Therefore, the aim is to choose a material which has the nearest thermal properties to the oral tissues in the region of its use.

Specific heat capacity plays a major role in melting and casting procedures, since it determines the total amount of heat that should be applied to raise temperature of the metal to its melting point.

In case of metal restorations, the coefficient of expansion should approach that of enamel and dentin, so that any change in temperature within the mouth does not cause different dimensional change between the tooth and the restoration.

ELECTRICAL PROPERTIES

Electricity, in simple words is the flow of electrons across an electron gradient. And since metals contain free electrons, it becomes imperative to discuss the electrical properties of material.

The ability of a material to conduct an electric current across it is its **electrical conductivity.** Resistance to the flow of electric current is **electrical resisitivity.**

The conductivity of different materials is different. This implies that when dis-similar metals are placed in opposition, a flow of electric current can occur between the metals. If an electrolyte solution is present between the metals to enable the flow of electrons a complete electric circuit is formed and flow of electric current occurs. This phenomenon is called **Galvanism** and the current which flows is the **Galvanic current.**

The Galvanic current with saliva as the electrolyte solution causes degradation of the material, which is called **Corrosion.**

Galvanic Cell

A Galvanic Cell has 4 Components :

1. Anode :

This is where oxidation takes place by loss of electrons from the metal atom. As a result, degradation occurs at the Anode.

2. Cathode :

This is the electrode where Reduction occurs, by consumption of electrons produced at the Anode. Metal ions are removed from solution to form metal atoms.

3. External Circuit :

It is the pathway to carry electrons from the Anode to the Cathode.

4. Electrolyte Solution :

It is a weak electrolyte solution which enables dissolution at the Anode.

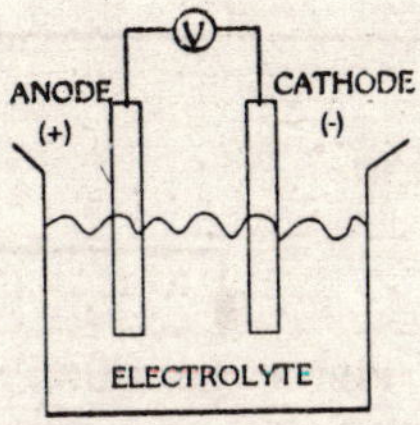

When two dissimilar metals are present, it is important to know which metal will undergo corrosion, in other words, which will function as the Anode. This is given by Electro Motive Force (EMF Series). The EMF series is nothing but a comparision of the solubility of different metals ,when kept in a standard electrolyte solution.

The ability of a material to undergo dissolution in a standard electrolyte solution is measured by keeping hydrogen as the reference elecrode. It is given an arbitrary value of zero.

There can be 2 possibilities when placing a metal specimen in such an experimental set up :

1. The metal specimen can undergo dissolution, by oxidation reaction. This will cause loss of metal substance. Such metals are given a negative EMF value.
2. The metal specimen can cause deposition of metal atoms on it by reduction, and thus increase its mass. Such metals are given a positive EMF Value.

Thus the metal with the highest negative value will undergo maximum corrosion. Hence with the EMF series, we can know which metal will corrode, when placed with a dissimilar metal in the oral cavity. However, the EMF series cannot quantify corrosion. This is because the electrolyte solution composition and concentration also determine the dissolution of metals.

Galvanism can occur even in a single isolated restoration, where heterogenicity of the metal or the electrolyte solution cause formation of galvanic cell.

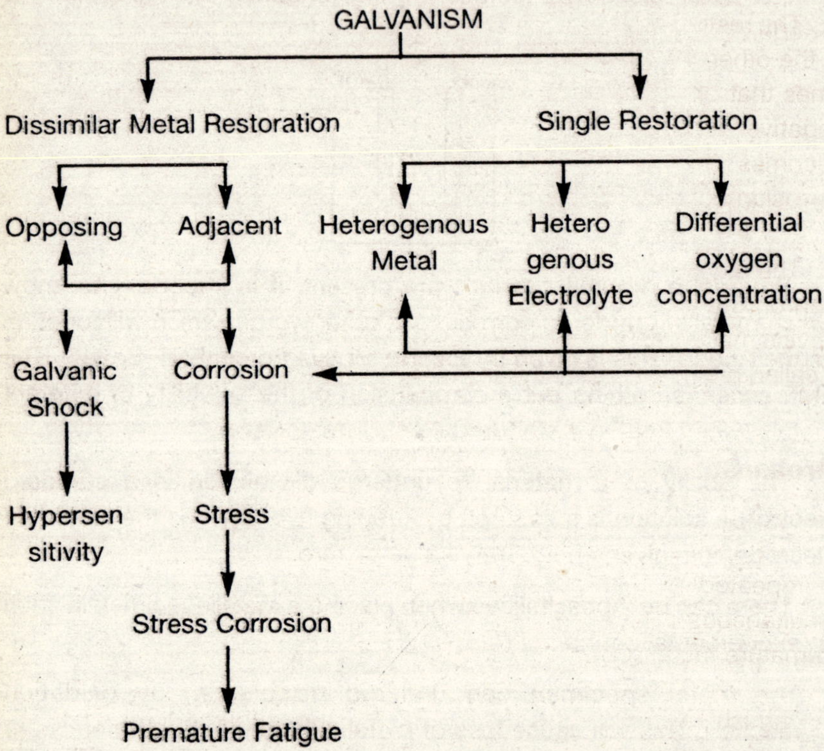

How does Galvanism arise in a single restoration.

If the metal is an alloy (Eutectic or Peritectic), there exists Heterogenicity in the metal. The different constituent metals set up a galvanic cell. Even a solid solution alloy is not perfectly homogenous.

In the oral cavity, the electrolytic composition of saliva varies in different areas. Heterogenicity of the electrolyte solution (ie. saliva) will set up a galvanic cell.

The restoration contacts saliva at one surface and the dentinal fluid at the other. The Chloride (Cl^-) concentration of dentinal fluid is seven times that of saliva, thus making the dentinal end of the restoration a negative terminal with respect to the surface (which obviously becomes the Anode). Hence a galvanic cell is established and corrosion occurs.

The oxygen concentration in the crevices of the restoration is less than on the exposed surface of metal. The absence of oxygen in the crevice makes it behave like an anode, where corrosion will occur. This is called crevice corrosion or concentration cell corrosion.

Stress Corrosion

The accumulation of stress in dental restoration or appliance due to repeated removal and insertion, or cold working, along with simultaneous corrosion that occurs in the oral environment can cause premature fatigue of the material. This is called stress corrosion.

Tarnish occurs on the surface of the metal when a non metalic substance reacts with it in the absence of an electrolyte solution.

Since the same electrons determine the thermal and electric properties of the material, these two properties should be dealt with together. An increase in temperature increases the electrical conductivity, and the flow of current through a material increases its temperature.

CONCLUSION

There are many more properties, the understanding of which is essential for the proper utilisation of the materials. This chapter aimed at explaining a few important problems in a simple way for the reader to understand it.

THE DECLINE OF GOLD RESTORATIONS

Karthikeyan K.S.

INTRODUCTION :

Right from prehistoric times, mankind has been fascinated by gold. As elemental gold was not only found in the free state in nature, but also in combination with lead or copper sulfide, it was extracted easily and used extensively in jewellery, medicine and dentistry. Being the most malleable and ductile material, its manipulation is easy, working instruments and equipment needed are simple and minimal. In the rigourous conditions of wet oral environment, the high corrosion and tarnish resistance of gold is a boon. It was estimated that approximately one lakh nine thousand kilograms of gold were used in dentistry per year, prior to 1970. This was roughly seven percent of the total gold consumed per year in all fields, then. But, with the spiralling price of gold in the early seventies, the usage of gold in dentistry diminished. The price of gold increased tenfold and remains at that level with minimal periodical fluctuations. Such steep increase has been the beginning of the decline of gold restorations in dentistry.

USE OF GOLD IN EARLIER TIMES :

Historically, gold use was restricted to prosthetic dentistry and periodontia during the earlier period. Replacement of one or more teeth banded with existing natural teeth, or use of gold wires to splint natural teeth were the norm. Covering natural teeth with gold bands was also done as a status enhancement measure. Direct gold fillings were done by Giovanni Arcolani almost five hundred years ago. Gold castings were done in the beginning of twentieth century.

USE OF GOLD IN MODERN TIMES :

In modern dentistry, gold is one of the few metals to be used in the elemental form. Pure cohesive gold is used as a restorative material. The gold has to be 99.9.% pure (999 fine or 24 carat) and free from any contaminants. The gold used as a direct filling could be in the form of foil, electrolytic precipitate of mat gold, powdered gold or alloyed gold. One type of alloyed gold is where calcium is added upto 0.1%, to increase the strength. In another type of alloyed gold, a platinum foil is interposed between two gold foils and bonded by a cladding process and this increases the strength of the material. Sometimes silver is also alloyed to gold. Conventional gold beating (forging, resulting in mechanical thickness reduction) is used for preparing the fibrous gold foil and electrolytic precipitation is done for manufacturing the crystalline mat gold that is available as strips. Gold foil, in addition to being supplied as sheets are also supplied in vaious sizes and shapes, as cylinders, ropes or pellets. Chemically or electrolytically precipitated gold powder is also used as a direct filling gold. Powdered gold is mixed with wax for better cohesion and wrapped in a foil for easier handling. The wax is to be burnt out during degassing procedure and gold compacted in the cavity. Recently developed E-Z gold and stopfgold are claimed to be superior in their handling properties and strength.

Alloys of gold are widely used in the cast form than the wrought form. Development of Taggart's technique of casting by lost wax process in the beginning of this century gave an impetus to use of alloyed gold as a cast restration. Crowns, inlays, onlays, bridges, partial denture bases and retentive clamps are made from alloyed gold. Reinforcement of softer gold is done by adding copper, palladium and silver. Judicious alterations in the composition of various metals resulted in different types of alloys suitable for diverse situations. Gold formed the major ingredient (between 69 and83%) of these alloys. Increase in price of gold resulted in substitution with other cheaper noble metals (mainly palladium) in the place of gold and low gold alloys resulted. Such low gold alloys, non gold alloys of palladium - silver or base metal alloys form the basis for cast restorations nowadays rather than high gold casting alloys.

Whenever steel pins are used for enhancing the retention of restoration, there is a possibility of their corrosion in the long run and their failure. To overcome this disadvantage, electroplating of the pin is done with gold. Such gold plated pins offer better corrosion resistance. These gold plated pins are useful for intra orally made incrementally added restorations like silver amalgam or composite resins. For cast restorations, parallel pin channels are made and plastic pins could be inserted into them to unite with the wax pattern and subsequently the cast gold pins are the extensions of the casting. If increased strength of the gold pins is desired, swaged gold smooth pins are inserted to the pin channels and they become extensions of the wax pattern to be invested. After investing and wax elimination, lower part of the swaged pins are buried in the investment and upper part of the swaged gold pins extending into the mould space. When molten gold alloy enters the mould, it unites with the swaged gold alloy pin.

Whenever gross destruction of crown structure has taken place and adequate core is not present to provide the base for the crown preparation, a cast post and core is done. Such custom made preparation done with gold alloy offers the advantages of strength and reinforcement. Preformed wrought gold posts are also available in various sizes and after selecting a suitable one, gold core can be cast onto it.

Wax forms are available in the shapes of clasps & occlusal rests for preparing the pattern for cast gold clasps and occlusal rests. Such clasps will be part of partial denture gold alloy denture bases. Instead, wrought wires could also be custom made into clasps, to unite with the cast gold denture base.

To avoid excessive wear of the occlusal surfaces of artificial dentures, occlusal portions alone are made of cast gold alloy which is connected by mechanical means to the underlying acrylic teeth and denture base. This prevents the rapid wear of the acrylic teeth during function in heavy biters.

Gold - Silver - Copper alloy wrought wires and Gold - platinum - palladium wrought wires are also available in different sizes. They are used for orthodontic appliances. However, they are not superior to stainless steel wires. The compsition of these gold alloy wires can vary among the different types. The metals used in these alloys are gold, palladium, platinum, silver, copper and traces of nickel and zinc. There are eight types of alloy compositions in this category.

Attaining a moisture free area in the periapex is a difficult task. But this is also obtained and direct filling gold is used as a retrograde filling material, following apicectomy.

When complete surgical closure of an oro antral fistula is not possible, attempts are made to close the defect with foils.

In cases of palatal erosion, palatal gold veneers are made with minimal or no tooth preparation.

ADVANTAGES OF GOLD RESTORATIONS :

The resons for the above mentioned divrse usage of gold are the unique properties that are advantageous to the dental surgeon. A restoration from which no ingredient leaches out to irritate the pulp or periodontium is a great advantage. Gold is chemically inert and is highly biocompatiable. Allergy to gold is very rare. Another advantage of gold is its ability to take up high polish and retain it. Such smooth surfaces do not cause any physical irritation to tissues contacting it and the smooth surface is unfavourable for plaque accumulation. Alloyed gold has adequate strength to withstand the masticatory load, especially types II, III and IV high gold alloys. Even direct filling gold becomes harder because of cold working and surface burnishing. Yet another advantage of gold is its ability to be burnished. The high malleability and ductility permits burnishing the restoration at the beveled margin to reduce the marginal leakage. For cast restorations, burnishing prevents the exposure of the luting cement.

The high wear resistance of the gold restoration demarcate it as a permanent restoration and unlike porcelain, it does not cause excessive wear of the oppsite natural tooth. Gold is insoluble in oral fluids and there is neither structural loss nor systemic toxicity on this account. Gold has low modulus of elasticity and the clasps made out of them can spring out of undercuts without difficulty. For bonding with porcelain, suitable gold alloys are available with compatible fusion and firing temperatures, compatible coefficient of thermal expansion and ability to chemically bond with porcelain through tin oxide or indium oxide. For making gold restorations, simple instruments and laboratory equipment will suffice and that is an advantage. Gold restorations are time tested, unlike the recently developed Castable ceramics, CAD CAM porcelain, Hiceram or Composites.

THE CAUSES FOR REDUCTION IN GOLD USE :

The numrous advantages of gold restorations are outweighed by the few disadvantages that co-exist and this has led to the diminishing use of gold restorations. Let us examine the various factors that have contributed to the downfall of gold restorations. These factors could be subdivided into (A) Patient factors (B) Operator factors (C) Material factors and (D) Laboratory factors.

(A) Factors connected with the patient :

1. Higher cost : As far as the patient is concerned, cost of the treatment plays an important role in decision making. If cheaper alternatives are available, many patients would prefer that.

2. Comfort : If direct filling gold is to be given as a restoration, the prolonged period for which the mouth is to be kept open, with the rubber dam in position might be too tiring for the patient. If open flame degassing is done, patient always has an apprehension of possible thermal burn to the tooth or the soft tissues. If malletting is used for compaction, patient might be annoyed by the jarring effect that might be present.

3. Necessity of extra visits : If cast gold restorations are planned, the patient is requested to visit the dental clinic atleast twice. Many patients would prefer to have a single sitting restoration as they consider themselves to be too busy to spare time for such mundane activity as a dental visit. Many patients want maximum dentistry in minimum time. (preferably in a single visit)

4. Aesthetics :The sense of appreciation of beauty varies between different cultures and from time to time. It is a matter of individual preference and psychological factors play a predominant role. Gold, with its powerful yellowish hue, is always associated with richeness and in the earlier days, people preferred to have an anterior gold crown as a status symbol. But presently people prefer to have a restoration that completely merges with its surroundings and is unnoticeable. Most patients prefer to display the gold as jewellery than a restoration.

5. Galvanic pain : A patient who has heard about or experienced galvanic pain will definitely want to avoid it all cost. He might not be convinced about the lesser corrodability of gold filling. He would prefer to do without the gold filling rather than changing the numerous amalgam fillings already present.

6. Allergy :The occurence of gold allergy is extermely rare, but if present, the patient would want an alternative restoration. No dental surgeon will force any patient to have a gold restoration, if he suspects that the patient might be allergic to gold.

7. Fear about personal safety : Histroy is full of instances of cruelty perpetuated by one race over another. Mass killings, ethnic cleansing and genocides have taken place in all parts of the globe. Jewellery in possession of the vanquished were seized by the victors and even teeth with gold restorations were brutally plucked out from living and dead victims of the concentration camps. There is no guarantee that such atrocities will not be repeated as the human greed and avarice remain unabated. May be the patient, in his fear of personal safety, preferring to avoid gold restorations is justified in his action!

(B) Factors related with the operators :

1. Necessity of higher skill : For direct filling gold restorations, more patience, greater stamina and better skill of the operator are needed. Each increment of gold should be carefully placed and meticulously condensed to avoid voids and defects. Lack of experience and exposure to direct filling gold fillings make a dental surgeon feel inadequate to perform such a restoration. This is only the fear of the unknown. With constant practice, the dental surgeon can develop the required skill for any procedure. Lack of training in handling direct gold fillings in dental colleges could be cited as the only reason for not aquiring the required skill.

2. Lure of cosmetic dentistry : Most dental surgeons prefer to do restorations that blend with the natural tooth substance, thereby merging with the surroundings. This is in accord with the old adage, 'the greatest art is to conceal art'. Such invisiable restorations are preferred by patients also. Though the currently available tooth coloured restorations have their own disadvandages and drawbacks, they are used preferentially in all situations. The advantages of gold restoratious are not highlighted by the dental surgeons atleast in situations favouring it and because of its colour, gold is rejected.

3. Need for more chairside time : Practice management has become an exact science and dental surgeons are taught by management experts how to cut costs and save precious chairside time for treating more patients. In search for greater profits, may be dental surgery has been converted from a profession to a commercial enterprise. Such dehumanisation of dentistry, to make as much money as possible in the available time, might endanger the confidence a patient has in his dentist. Earning profits and hoping to get better returns on the investment are no crime. The same could be achieved by spending more chairside time with the patient and charging more, rather than denying a better restoration merely because it involves more chairside time. If gold restoration is indicated in any situation, the dental surgeon should preferably give it, in spite of the increased chairside time.

4. Possible pulpal & periodontal damage : For direct filling gold restorations, excessive condensation forces might cause pulpal and / or periodontal damage. However, normal hand pressure of 10 to 15 pounds does not cause any irreversible pulpal or periodontal changes.

5. Possible damage to enamal margins : Careless use of condensor tips while doing a direct filling gold may break the enamel margin and that should be avoided. Always, a piece of gold should be present between the condenser tip and the tooth substance to avoid damage to the tooth. Even while condersing gold in the deeper part of the covity, care should be taken that the shank of the condenser does not inadvertently impinge on the enamal margin, cracking or fracturing it. This could be one of the fears of the operator that prevents him use the direct filling gold.

6. Extra care during degassing : Correct desorbing should be done to obtain optimum results. Gold, a noble metal, does not react with its surroundings. But intentional surface coating of ammonia to prevent accidental contamination with other tenacious chemicals like sulphur, phosphorous and chlorine, should be removed before condensation. Degassing could be done either with an open flame by directly flaming the gold, over a mica tray kept above a flame or in an electric annealer. Whichever method is used, absolute cleanliness is a prerequiste. Even a match stick should not be lit in the presence of direct filling gold, for the possibility of contamination of gold by sulphur and phosphorous fumes. As an open flame, even a clean Bunsen flame could be used, though an acetone free alcohol flame is preferred. The correct degassing procedure should be followed and the electric annealer should be kept at the temperature between 340°C & 370°C. Powdered gold with a wax or organic binder, wrapped in a gold foil, should be held above the flame, allowed to catch fire, the binder should burn out and the gold should turn cherry red in colour. Such exacting procedure should be carefully followed. During desorbing, underheating will not remove all the contaminants and there will be incomplete cohesion. Overheating can lead to over sintering and gold will become brittle and will not cohere.

7. Suspicion about pilferage : When dental surgeon does not do the casting procedure himself and has to depend upon another individual to do the gold casting, there will always be a suspicion about the quality of gold used for the casting. Though almost all the technicians involved may be scrupulously honest, the possibility of a dishonest individual stealing gold (because of its high cost) might deter a dental surgeon from using gold restorations.

(C) Factors connected with the material :

1. Economy : A low gold alloy (containing 46% of gold, 40% of silver, 6% of palladium and 6% of copper) is cheaper by 30% than a conventional high gold alloy. Another low gold alloy (containing 15% gold, 45% silver, 25% palladium and 14% copper) is cheaper by 45% than a conventional high gold alloy. A silver - palladium alloy (70 : 25) costs only 10% of the price of conventional high gold alloy, so availability of cheaper substitutes with clinical acceptability has reduced the usage of conventional high gold alloys.

2. Non-availability of instruments & equipment : Not only in India, but also in America there appears to be difficulties in obtaining equipment and materials for direct filling gold. Lambert laments that there is continuing pressure to minimize or eliminate the direct gold restoration from the dental curriculum in U.S.A. and this makes it impossible or extrmely difficult for operative faculty to purchase mechanical condensers for student use. The declining demand might have made the manufacture of mechanical condensers less profitable.

3. Lack of indigenous manufacture of dental gold : Though India is the largest consumer of gold in the world, there is no local manufacture & distribution of direct filling gold or cast gold alloys. Whatever gold restorations are done in India, It is only done with imported gold that adds up to the cost or with jewellery gold, which is inferior in properties.

4. ***High thermal conductivity :*** The thermal conductivity of gold restorations is approximately 400 times that of the natural tooth. However, this might not be very influencial for the reduced use of gold restorations, as direct filling gold is not given for deep cavities and in a deep inlay cavity, a thermal insulating base is invariably given.

5. ***Possible galvanic effect :*** Electrode potential of a metal indicates its ability to go into ionic solution in the presence of an electrolytic media. The presence of two dissimilar metals connected together in an electrolytic media results in passage of electric current from the metal with more negative potential to the metal with more positive potential, thereby causing electrochemical corrosion of the more electronegative metal.

6. ***Softness of pure gold :*** 100% pure gold is only as hard as lead. Alloying with other elements like copper, silver, palladium, platinum, iridium, calcium etc. increases the strength of gold. Strength of pure direct filling gold is also increased by the malletting, condensing and finishing of direct gold restorations. Such increase in strength is due to atomic remodelling called strain hardening, brought by cold working.

7. ***Higher density of gold alloys :*** The density of gold is 19.3 gms/c.c. and is almost double that of chrome - cobalt alloys. This means, for a given volume of restoration, not only the base metal alloy will be cheaper, but also lighter and hence more comfortable, to the patient.

8. ***Colour of the gold :*** Almost all the metals barring gold and copper are white or resembling it. Addition of silver, platinum, palladium etc. tend to overcome the yellow or red colour of gold or copper and the alloy appears whitish. However, addition of no metal is capable of alterning the colour of gold to the colour of tooth.

9. ***Evolution of newer materials :*** Science can never be static. There will always be never inventions and improvements and

changes are inevitable. Though the human mind finds comfort with the established and the conventional, newer methods and materials should be tried, initially for evaluation, and if found sutable, for betterment of the professional service. If a newer material is found superior to gold restorations, it should readily be accepted. However, the currently available alternatives, though superior to gold restorations in a property or two, are definitely inferior in other respects.

(D) Factors Related to laboratory Processing :

Fabrication of cast gold restorations is an exacting technique. Errors at any stage of processing may lead to failure of restoration.

1. Failure to ensure effective shrinkage compensation : Manufacturers are expected to provide the accurate information regarding the shrinkage percentage of inlay wax and the casting alloy as well as the percentage of expansion of the investment. When such information is not provided, planning the required mould expansion might be more of guesswork and conjecture and this can result in an oversized or undersized restoration.

2. Failure to immediately confine wax pattern in investment : Inlay wax patterns, upon storage, tend to release the accumulated stresses and this can lead to alteration in its shape.

3. Using an investment with greater setting expansion : An inlay wax pattern invested immediately can also undergo distortion due to uneven pull in areas of different thickness of wax pattern due to setting expansion. The thinner gingival portion could be forced apart by the mould expansion than the thicker occlusal postion.

4. Wrong direction of sprue former attachment : When a sprue former is attached perpendicular to a floor or wall, the molten alloy tends to hit the same spot repeatedly before flowing to other portions of the mould, thereby elevating the temperature of the mould at that spot to higher levels, creating a hot spot. Because of the rise in temperature, the alloy near the hot spot will be the last to solidify, resulting in suckback porosity. Not flaring the sprue former at the site of attachemnt will also cause suckback porosity.

5. Excessive distance between the pattern & casting ring : Having more than 6 millimeters of back–up investment while using gypsum bonded investment and more than 3 millimeters while using phosphate bonded investment could prevent easy escape of trapped air from within the mould space and this can result in back pressure porosity.

6. Non use of vents for denser investments : In Brumfield's method of venting, a 14 gauge diameter wax rod isattached to the periphery of the crucible former base and the free end is bent around the pattern and brought to 3 m.m. short of the fitting surface of the pattern. Direct venting could also be used with a16 gauge wax rod.

7. Inadequacy in size and location of reservoir : Reservoirs smaller than the bulkiest portion of the pattern or larger reservoirs positioned more than two millimetres above the wax patterns might not serve their purpose of shinkage compensation and porosity might result.

8. Using an investment with large particle size : Larger particle size of the investment prevents closer adaptation with the wax patterns & results in rougher castings.

9. Failure to use vacuum investing : There is a possibility of air bubble entrapment and if it occurs in a critical part of the casting may result in poor fit, even after removable of the nodule.

10. Inadequate care during manual investing : Failure to use mechanical mixing technique and not using a vibrator during investing may also result in air entrapment. While using a single investment technique, chances of air bubble entrapment is higher.

11. Careless removal of sprue former : During removal of sprue former, if sufficient care is not taken, bits of investment can fall into the mould and that could result in a deficient casting.

12. Faster rate of heating the mould : The rate of heating should be about 10°cto 12° C / minute. If it is much higher than this, water is not removed gradually and development of steam pockets in the mould can crack the investment which might be seen as fin formation incasting.

13. Inadequate heating of mould : When hygroscopic expansion is the primary mode of shinkage compensation, the mould is heated only upto 468°C. Even if the temperature is held at this temperature for an hour or hour and a half, complete elimination of carbon residues might not occur and this can result in gaseous porosity in casting or a tenacious black discolouration of casting.

14. Inadequate air circulation during wax elimination : When an investment ring is kept in a furnace for wax elimination, it is usually kept initially with the crucible side down to permit the gravitational flow of the molten wax to come out. After about twenty minutes, the ring position is reversed to have the crucible side up. The furance door is also kept open to have more air circulation to ensure complete burn out of carbon residues. This is especially useful for hygroscopic techniques.

15. Excessive heating of the mould : Too long a time used for heating the mould, or heating the mould to a very high temperature than indicated can result in craking or crumbling of the investment mould surface resulting in a rough casting. Sulphur gases evolved from disintegrated investment can also cause black discolouration.

16. Inadequate heating of alloy : This can result in higher viscosity of the molten alloy and may result in an incomplete casting.

17. Failure to provide a reducing atmosphere during melting of alloy: Showing the oxidizing zone over the alloy or failure to use a charcoal crucible to create a reducing atmosphere may permit the molten silver and copper to absorb oxygen and hydrogen and releasing than upon solidification. Such gas inclusion porosities are definitely determental to the castings.

18. Excessive heating of the alloy : Usually the alloys are heated to about 50°C higher than the higher limit of their melting range. If excessive heating is done, the overheated alloy could attack the investment and a rough casting might result. Moreover, too much difference in mould - melt temperature can result in suck back porosity.

19. Non-use of electrically driven casting machine : For faster initial acceleration of the arms of the casting machine, an electrically driven casting machine is superior to spring activated casting machine. Among the spring activated casting machines also, a heavy duty spring provides better rate of intial acceleration than a lighter spring.

20. Excessive casting pressure : More than 20 psi air pressure ormore than five turns ofspring activation in a centrifugal casting machine can damage thesurface of the moulddue to too high a force of the molten alloy and result in a rough casting. The excessive force of impact of molten alloy could also break a vulnerable portion of the investment mould.

The above mentioned factors involved in the laboratory processing techniques highlight the technique sensititivity of the cast gold restorations and may be these are some of the inhibiting factors for the widespread use of gold restoration.

NEWER INTRODUCTIONS :

To enthuse young dental surgeons into using direct filling gold restorations, newer materials and easier condensation techniques are developed. The introduction of E-Z gold and stopfgold are the steps in the steps in that direction. E-Z gold is a type of powdered gold with less than 0.01% organic wax that could be hand condensed like a stiff amalgam but the material is more cohesive than gold foil. Manipulation of the material is claimed to be easy.

Stopfgold is a chemically precipitated gold powder that underwent a milling process after precipitation. The particles are then loosely sintered together and cut into strips 3 millimetres wide and 40 millimetres in length and available in three different thicknesses of 0.7 m.m. 1 m.m. and 1.5 m.m. microscopically the material consists of flat polygonal platelets with a diameter of 25 to 75 micrometres and thickness of 1.5 m.m. Hand condensation is considered to produce a clinically satisfactory restoration, and is claimed to be easier to condence than Electralloy. The disadvantage of this material is said to be its cost that is 75% more than other forms of granular gold. But still, it is claimed to cost approximately only about Rs. 600/- for an average sized class V cavity.

The current attempts are to develop gold with better cohesive properties so that hand condensation will be able to produce a satisfactory restoration. Complicated condensing gadgets are slowly eased out of the profession.

CONCLUSION :

There is definitely a decline in the use of gold in dentistry and price rise is not the only reason for it. Patient's preference for tooth coloured restorations, tremendous improvements in material science with evolution of newer options, difficulty in procuring gold condensing instruments and equipment and lack of training for dental surgeon have all contributed to the decline. The newer developments in powdered gold and the suggested easier condensation techniques appear far too inadequate to rekindle interest in use of gold. To imagine that gold will occupy its rightful place as the most permanent restoration and will widely be used, appears to be only wishful thinking. Generally it appears that it is difficult to arrest the decline of use of gold restoration and that is the sad truth.

BONDING

Lakshmi Narayanan L.

TERMINOLOGY

Atom : Any of the smallest particles of an element that combine with similar particles of other elements to produce compounds.

In other words, a tiny particle of anything.

Adhesion : The force that holds together the molecules of unlike substances whose surfaces are in contact.

Bond : Any thing that binds, fastens or restrain.

Cohesion: The force by which the molecules of a substance are held together.

Dipole : Any system having two equal but opposite electric charges or magnetic poles separated by a very small distance.

Energy : Inherent power, capcity for vigorous action.

Force : The cause, or agent that puts an object at rest into motion or alters the motion of moving object.

Molecule : Molecules of elements consist of one atom or two or more similar atoms. (Those of compounds consists of two or more different atoms)

Polarity : The condition of being positive or negative with respect to some reference point or object.

Surface Tension : A property of liquids in which the exposed surface tends to contact to the smallest possible area because of unequal molecular cohesive forces near the surface. Measured by force/unit of length.

INTRODUCTION :

All materials are built up trom atoms and molecules, so it is not really surprising that there is a close relationship between the atomic structure of a material and its properties.

The atoms combine to determine the microstructure of the solid and as a consequence determine its properties. When two atoms are brought together they may link to form a molecule, any bond that form are called PRIMARY BONDS. The controlling factor in bond formation is ENERGY and a bond will only form if it results in a lowering of the total energy of atoms being joined, that is if the total energy of the molecule is less than the sum of the energies of the separate atoms, irrespective of the type of bond being formed.

The conditions under which the atoms bond together, depend upon the electron configurations which completely determine their chemical reactivity. The more stable the electron configuration, the less reactive the atom. This is caused by having complete outermost electron orbitals with no opportunity for more electrons to join the atom and no spare or loose electrons to leave the atom. The atoms of some elements have gaps for electrons in their outermost orbits whereas the atoms of other elements have spare electrons in their outermost orbits. By combining with each other these two different types of atoms can both acheive complete outermost orbitals. The formation of bonds therefore involves only the outermost valence electrons. The forces that hold atoms together are called cohesive forces. These **INTERATOMIC BONDS** may be classified as Primary or Secondary. The strength of these bonds as well as their ability to reform after breakage determines the physical properties of the material.

TYPE OF BONDS:

PRIMARY ATOMIC BONDS - are of 3 types:

(i) Ionic (ii) Covalent (iii) Metallic

(i) Ionic : These are of the simple chemical type, resulting from mutual attraction of positive and negative charges, that is electron transfer from one element (positive) to another (negative). Ionic bonds result in crystals whose atomic configuration is based on charge balance. In dentistry, ionic bonding exist in certain crystalline phases of some dental materials such as gypsum and phosphate cements.

(ii) Covalent Bonds : This is the simplest and strongest bond, which arises when atoms share their electrons so that each electron shell achieves an inert structure. A typical characteristic of covalent bonds are their directional orientation. Covalent bonding occurs in many organic compounds such as dental resins, to which they link forming the backbone structure of hydrocarbon chairs.

(iii) Metallic Bonds: In this, atoms can easily donate electrons from their outer shell and form a gas of free electrons. The contribution of free electrons to this cloud results in the formation of positive ions that can be neutralised by acquiring new valence electrons from adjacent atoms (eg.gold). Because of their ability to donate and recover electrons, atoms in a metal crystal exist as clusters of positve metal ions surrounded by a gas of electrons. This is responsible for the excellent electrical and thermal conductivity of metals and also for their ability to deform plastically.

INTERATOMIC SECONDARY BONDS:

In contrast with primary bonds, secondary bonds do not share electrons. Instead charge variations among molecules or atomic groups induce power forces that attract the molecule. A consequence of sharing of electrons by two or more atomic nuclei is that, electrons wil spend a disproportionate longer time in one particular position. The effect of this is that one end of the molecule may acquire a slight positive charge and the other end a slight negative charge resulting in an electric imbalance known as **ELECTRIC DIPOLE.** These dipoles allow molecules to interact with one another and to form weak bonds called **VANDER WAALS BONDS** eg. In a symmetric molecule, such of which occurs in an inert gas, the electronic field is constantly fluctuating.

Normally, the electrons of the atoms are distributed equally around the nucleus and produce an electrostatic field around the atom. This field may fluctuate so that its charge becomes momentarily positive and negative. A fluctuating dipole is thus created that wil attract other similar dipoles.

Such interatomic forces are weak and these are called Vander waals forces, which forms the basis of dipole attraction.

Regardless of the type of matter, there is a limiting factor that prevents the atoms or molecules from approaching each other too closely, that is the distance between the center of an atom and that of its neighbour is limited to the diameter of atoms involved. If the atoms approach too closely, they are repelled from each other by their electron charges. On the other hand, forces of attraction tend to draw the atoms together. The position of which these forces of repulsion and attraction become equal in magnitude is the equilibrium position of the atoms. Conditions of equilibrium are usually described in terms of energy (or) interatomic energy.

As the resultant force approaches zero the energy decreases. The energy finally reaches a minimum when the resultant force becomes zero. Thereafter the energy increases rapidly because the resultant repulsive forces increases rapidly with little change in interatomic distance. Of the bonds, covalent bonds tend to be the strongest having bond energy of 6.3 Ev-4 followd by ionic bond ranging from 4.2 to 3.2 and finally the metallic bonds with energy ranging rom 2.3 to .2 for mercury. So mercury has the very low bond energy, giving a bond that is not strong enough to hold the atoms in place at room temperature resulting in mercury's liquidity at this temperature. An example of how secondary bonding forms the basis of the molecular attraction in molecular solids is Ice.

Covalent solids consisting of a single element find to be very rare. Covalent bonds are more usually formed between dissimilar elements. The electron orbitals overlap and the electrons are shared, resulting in a filled orbital which is very stable. Most elements which join by covalent bonding tend to be gases or liquids - Eg. water, oxygen and hydrogen. For the water to solidify at 0°C there must be some additional attraction between the water molecules other than covalent bond, something must hold these molecules together, it is not primary bond but secondary bond (ie) Vander waals bond (ie) Dipole attraction. The Vander waals forces are weaker than primary bonding because they are inter-molecular rather than intra-molecular.

ADHESION:

There are now many materials that we wish to BOND TO ENAMEL AND DENTINE and to each other. Numerous adhesives have been developed, such adhesives include composite resins, glass ionomer cements and dentine bonding agents. Adhesion can be defined as the force that binds two dissimilar materials together when they are brought into intimate contact. When there is contact between two solid surfaces, at an atomic level, surfaces are rough so, contact is achieved at the lips of asperities. When the solid and liquid are brought in contact there is a good adhesion, it is due to liquids ability to make intimate contact with the solid over a large surface area.

So a strong bond can be created only in the case of intimate molecular contact. For a good bond, the distance between the interacting molecules must be less than 0.0007 microns and adhesion is virtually impossible for two solid surfaces. Inorder to overcome this, we use a third substance usually in a fluid or semi fluid state, to act as an Intermediary. For adhesion to exist, the surface must be attracted to one another at their interface. Considering the SURFACE ENERGY, the energy at the surface of a solid is greater than that of its interior.

For example taking into account the space lattice, inside the lattice all the atoms are equally attaracted to each other. The interatomic distances are equal and the energy is minimal. At the surface of the lattice, the energy is greater because the outermost atoms are not equally attracted in all directions. The surface atoms of a solid tend to form bonds to other atoms that are in close proximity to the surface and thus reduce the surface energy of the solid. Eg. reduced by any surface impurity such as adsorbed gas or an oxide.

When there is greater surface energy, there is greater capacity for adhesion. Other example which can lower the surface energy is a film water, even one molecule thickness on the surface of the solid may lower the surface energy of the adherend and prevent any wetting by the adhesive. Some substance itself has a very low surface energy. Eg. Teflon - Polytetrafluroethylene.

Thus a low surface energy liquid will readily spread over a high surface energy substrate because the surface of the substrate is replaced by a surface with a lower surface energy. Teflon has a very low surface energy making it difficult to find liquids with lower surface energy that could wet it successfully. Transferring this information to the clinical setting. It is found that fluoride treated enamel surface retains less plaque because of a decrease in surface energy. Thus fluoride products may be effective in reducing dental caries by providing a tooth surface that stays cleaner over a longer period. Similarly because of the higher surface energy of many restorative materials compared with that of tooth, there is greater tendency for the surface and margins of the restoration to accumulate debris.

This may account for the relative high incidence of marginal caries seen around dental restoration. Regarding bonding to tooth surface, the greatest problem assoicated with this is water on the surface or saliva contamination. This water layer reduces the surface energy and thus may reduce the wetting of the adhesive restorative material. The inorganic components of tooth structure have a strong affinity for water. To remove water, the enamel and dentine would have to be heated to an unacceptable temperature which is not desirable.

So the dental adhesive must displace the water, react with it or wet the surface better than the water that is already present on and within the tooth structure. To enhance adhesive bonding, attempts are being made to use more hydrophilic resins that are not as sensitive to the presence of moisture as materials currently in use. The development of an adhesive approach to restorative dentistry has brought many advantages such as :

- Better aesthetics
- Conservation of tooth tissue.
- Improved crown strength
- Reduced potential for pulpal sensitivity.

The bonding systems that have studied include :

- The acid etch technique for bonding resins to enamel, now extensively used in placement of anterior and posterior composites, resin bonded bridges,venners and orthodontic brackets.

- The glass ionomer cements with their ability to bond to both enamel and dentine as direct adhesive restorations, act as dentine bonded bases under composite restorative materials, ceramic inlays and onlays.

ENAMEL BONDING:

The surface layer of enamel tends to have a higher organic content than the deeper layers and is protected by a layer of pellicle which is about 1 μm thick, (smear layer). When composite is placed on the tooth surface its major short coming is that they have no intrinsic adhesive qualities to tooth tissues as the resins are essentially non-polar.

So, the surface of the enamel can be modified by application of acid primers, thus making the surface of enamel more amenable to adhesive technique. Hence, the acid etch technique for bonding of composite restorative materials. So, enamel etchant's were developed.

This etching process modifies the surface by :

1) Increasing the surface roughness of the enamel.

2) It increasing the SURFACE ENERGY of the enamel by removing surface contaminations.

Increasing the surface area increases the bonding area. It is thus possible to bond to this surface by a process of micromechanical interlocking. Untreated enamel has a low surface energy (u) 28 $mJ.m^{-2}$ When it is treated by an acid, it increases the surface energy to 42$mJ.m^{-2}$, thus making the surface highly reactive. The resin will adapt well to this high surface energy surface as long as it is thoroughly dry. The drying process is equally critical to adhesion a perfectly dry enamel (since water is highly polar, the nonpolar resin will not adapt to a wet surface). The removal of surface hydroxyl group in the drying procedure will enhance the wettability of the resin on the surface and allow it to flow readily over the surface. It is important that the air-hose that is used for drying is free of any contaminants such as oil and water. Thus the acid etch bond to enamel is essentially mechanical.

DENTINE BONDING MECHANISM:

Primary role of dentine adhesive is to provide means for bonding hydrophobic composites to hydrophilic dentine. They act as an intermediary, and can be considered to be coupling agents in the sense that they are bifunctional and can combine with two distinctly different materials.

The general formula for the coupling agents in resin-based dentine adhesive is, Methacrylate group - Spacer group - Reactive group. Methacrylate group possess the double bond capable of bonding to the composite and provide a strong covalent bond. Spacer group must be able to provide the necessary flexibility to the coupling agent to enhance the potential for bonding of the reactive groups. If the molecule is excessively rigid, the ability of the reactive group to find a satisfactory conformational arrangement is at worst to limited to sites for bonding being available.

Reactive groups must be capable of chemically combining with the components of dentin in their organic or inorganic. They are polar pendent or end groups. The bond polarity is a consequence of asymmetrical electron distribution in the bond. Polar reactions occur as the result of attractive forces between positive and negative charges on the molecules. Thus the end groups on the coupling agent can combine with similar polar molecules in the dentine. Additionally, such a large molecule presumably could not readily diffuse into dentinal tubules and cause pulpal irritation. It could also act as a barrier to microleakage. We should be aware of the nature of the reactive group and whether its action is directed towards the inorganic (Ca-hydroxy apatite) or the organic (collagen or both components of dentin. Some of the agents are mixture of chemicals.

Classes of organic compounds that are thought to combine with the inorganic components of dentin are:-

1. Phosphates
2. Phenyl phosphates
3. Chlorophosphates
4. Chelating compounds
5. Carboxylic acid compounds

The reactive groups available in the principle organic component (collagen) in dentin are:

1. Amino
2. Amido
3. Hydroxyl
4. Carboxylate

These pendent groups on the long chain collagen molecule combine with the compounds containing reactive groups of:

1. Carboxylic acid chlorides
2. Carboxylic acid anhydrides
3. Isocyanates
4. Aldehydes

Bonding to dentin involves chemical reaction with the available reactive groups located in the organic as well as the inorganic. The resin based dentine bonding agents are believed to rely on a combination of physical attraction, mediated by the polar groups and the penetration in to the dentine, creating a molecular entanglement network. Essential components of dentine bonding agents are :

1. Primer
2. Coupling agent
3. Unfilled Resin

Primers-called dentine conditioners alter the surface appearence and characteristics of the dentine. Unfilled resin, reffered to as dentine sealer.

One of the major features distinguishing dentine bonding agents is the variety of dentine primers that can be used in some situation and in some, no primers at all. In the case of the later, the coupling agents directly bond to dentine. Bonding systems with acid primers modify the smear layer, that results in opening of the dentinal tubules and demineralises surface layer of dentine up to 4µm deep. The action of the coupling agent is to penetrate in to the demineralised dentine layer and create a molecular entanglement network. Problems associated with the use of dentine bonding agents are due to the nature of the dentine itself. Because of presence of water in the cut dentinal tissue. Dentine is hydrophilic where as most dentine adheives are hydrophobic.

So, the depth of penetration in these is aided by the use of a solvent carrier such as ethanol or acetone which is extremely effective at seeking out water and displacing it, carrying the coupling agents along as it goes. Thus, when these slovents are used, it makes the dentine surface more hydrophobic, thus preventing the resin from shrinking away from the walls with in the dentinal tubules and ensures the formation of the tightly fitting resin tag structure.

So these pull the adhesive in to the dentine with them.

In case of smear layer - EDTA or poly acrylic acid is used.

Other mode to increase bond strength of DBA are use of mordant ions. Ferric oxalate, Fe ions.This supplies a layer of ions for additional chelation. This is in addition to bonding which occurs with the calcium ions naturally present in the dentin. Disadvantage is that staining occurs at the interface between the restoration and the dentine thus resulting in adverse esthetic changes.

Mechanical bonding of bonding agent can be enhanced by widening of the dentinal tubles and thus deeper penetration of restorative material in to these tubules. These agents are pulpal irritants. Bonding to dentine involves certain factors namely :

1. Dentine 'actors
2. Tooth
3. Patient
4. Material

Dentine factors:

Includes microstructural features of the dentin involved with local adhesion, smear layer, dentinal tubule density, size and length, dentin sclerosis. Smear layer is partially porous and it dramatically reduces the fluid flow from the underlying dentinal tubules. It acts as a biological band aid reducing tooth post operative sensitivity. This layer affords a drier surface for adhesives involve procedures to remove or penetrate the smear layer. Adhesion is affected by wetness of the dentine, this in turn is related to the density and size of dentinal tubules. Tubules density is greatest near the pulp and tubules represent a much larger portion of the dentinal volume or around 28 volume % along the pulpal wall Vs 4 volume % at the DEJ.So this area has the greatest potential to immediately wet the cut dentinal surfaces.

Bond strengths in deep dentine generally are lower because of the interference of moisture from tubules. Newer dentine bonding systems include hydrophilic monomers that penetrate surface moisture and circumvent this problem.

Dentine sclerosis:

1. In response to caries, trauma or other stimuli, odontoblasts attempt to seal dentin by laying down a bridge of peritubular hydroxyapatite crystals. These sclerotic changes associated with aging may have an adverse effect on dentin bonding.

2. Tooth factors Include :

i. Lesion size and shape
ii. Enamel and dentine structure
iii. Tooth flexure
iv. Tooth location

Shallow, saucer shaped lesions lack insufficient surface area for adequate retention, precludes sufficient bulk of restorative material to resist deflection. This type of restoration appears to be particularly vulnerable to dislodgement during tooth flexture. Tooth flexture can be a contributer to the failure of dentinal adhesives. Eccentric forces on occlusal surface generate a critical flexture resulting in stress concentration in bonded areas. These flextural forces appear capable of debonding cervical restorations, especially those with out macro-mechanical retention.

Tooth location:

Greater cervical restoration failure occur in mandibular teeth related to difficulties with moisture control, or due to greater propensity for tooth flexture to occur in mandibular teeth, this again could occur as the result of lingual inclination of the crown and the smaller cross sectional area of mandibular teeth in the cervical area.

Patient factors:

History of bruxim or other traumatic occlusion produces greater occlusal stresses on their teeth. Clinical studies observed that, there is a link between the presence of occlusal stress and loss of cervical restoration retention.

Material factors:

At the outset,early improvements in dentin bonding agents had focussed on developing chemical bonds to tooth structure. But currently micro-mechanical bonding is emphasized.

Characteries and Bond Strengths of the First Five Generation of Bonding Systems

Bonding Generation	Characterists	Bond Strength to Dentin	Examples
Fifth	Single component Moist bonding No Mixing No sensitivity	>15Mpa	Printe & Bond 2.1. Syntac Single Compnent Bond 1 One Step Tenure Quick F
Fourth	Hybridization Total etch Little sensitivity	>15Mpa	All Bond II Pro Bond Tenure Bond It Syntac Scotchbond MP
Third	Two-component primer and adhesive system. Reduced sensitivity	10 Mpa	Prisma Universal Bond Tenure Scotchbond II
Second	Weak adhesive, require retentive preparations. Prone to water degradation	4.6 MPa	Bond Lite Scotchbond
First	Very weak	2 MPa	Cervident Consic bond

First generation DBA were designed for ionic bonding to hydroxyapatite or for covalent bonding to collagen. These materials were hydrophobic and were limited by the relative attachment strength of the smear layer to the underlying dentin. Bond strength was about 2 to 6 Mpa. New generation bonding agents procedures attempt to remove, penetrate or solublize the smear layer and then wet the underlying dentine with resin monomers that are more hydrophilic. Bond strength are decidedly improved by eliminating or penetrating the smear layer with mild organic acids.

However the dentin may be extensively demineralized and weakened depending upon the concentration of acid and exposure time. Stronger acids remove smear plugs and demineralize the intertubular dentin near the surface. After dentin conditioning, application of hydrophilic monomers penetrate the decalcified intertubular dentine and embed 1-5 μm of superficial dentine. This transitional zone called Hybrid layer, interpenetration zone or interdiffusion zone, appears to be the primary site for dential adhesion. Bonding strength ranaged from 12-22 Mpa. Hydrophilic systems seem to keep the collagen network open while penetrating it. Also polymerization shrinkage, water absorption of the overlying composite restoration also influence bond strength. More cervical retention failures are associated with a higher modulus composite that include macrofillers and a higher filler content. Where as macrofill composites with lower elastic moduli appear to flex in response to cervical deformation rather than debonding.

Amalgam Bonding Systems

They are used to bond amalgam to tooth structure, amalgam to amalgam or amalgam to other metal substrates.They require dual characteristics to achieve optimal wetting, Eg.dentai amalgam is strongly hydrophobic while dentine is hydrophilic. 4-META (4-methyloxyethyltrimelliticanhydride) is frequently used.This monomer molecule has hydrophobic and hydrophilic ends. The primary advantage for amalgam bonding agents is sealing of dentine. The bonding systems that produce a relatively thick (10-20μm) bonding agent layer permit the interlocking of microstructural features of amalgam during condensation and creates a strong interface. Adhesion of amalgam to weakened tooth structure, improves the over all resistance form of the restored tooth.

REFERENCES:

1. Phillips - Science of Dental Materials - Tenth Edition.
2. Clifford M.Sturdevant - The art and science of Operative Dentistry - Third Edition
3. Richard Van Noor - Introduction to Dental Materials (Published by Mosby in 1994
4. Glanz P.: On wettability and adhesiveness. Odontrev 20:1 (Suppl 17):1 1969

5. Nakapayashi N, Ashizawa M, Nakamura M: Identification of resin dentin hybrid layer in vital human dentin created in vivo, durable bonding to vital dentin. Quint Int 23:135 - 141,1992.

6. Joynt R.B,Davis E.L. Weizkowski.G et al. Dentin bonding agents and smear layer operative dent. 16:186-191,1991

7. George Freedman D.D.S, Fay goldstep D.D.S - Fifth generation bonding systems, State of the art in Adhesive Dentistry,Journal of Canadian Dental Association. Vol.63:No.6 June 1997.

8. Kanca J.Resin bonding to wet substrate 1. Bonding to dentin. Quintessence Intln. 23:39-41.1992

9. Bunocore MG : The use of adhesives in Dentistry. Springfield IL,Charles C thomas, 1975.

10. Bunocore MG : Journal of Dental Research 34:849,1995

11 Dr. N.S. Mohan Kumar, Dr. S. Balagopal Dr. L.Lakshmi Narayanan Smear layer - A review - JIDA, Jan 1998.

12. Dr. S. Balagopal - Tensile Bondstrength of three dentin adhesives - 1987.

AN INSIGHT ON BIO-COMPATIBILITY

Parameswaran A.

Compatible - Accordant, adaptable , agreeable, congeniality, empathy, harmony, congruent, congruous, consonant, in keeping, likeminded, reconcilable, suitable.

HISTORICAL PERSPECTIVE AND ORIGINAL USE OF THE DENTAL MATERIALS :

The use of foreign materials to replace or restore decayed or missing teeth is an ancient art. Even though tooth decay was recognized as a disease due to a vital organism earlier by the Chinese and the Sumarians, the technique of restoration of teeth was started only by 700 B.C. Etruscans replaced teeth missing through trauma, with human or animal substitutes using gold bands and wires. Such was the beginning of the earliest aesthetic treatments. Even a code of Hammurabi around 1700 BC was used for valuation of tooth in terms of its appearance and function, and was equated the value of a knocked out tooth to around the cost of a mina of silver. The dental procedures utilizing gold as crowns and bridges were followed by Romans after they conquered Etruscans. Many dentists advocated various dental procedures through the ages and during 100 AD Avicenna emphasised the importance of dental hygiene in medical practice which had influenced the medical practitioners for over 500 years.

In 1480 Avculans , a professor of medicine of Bologna described filling of teeth with gold foil. The earliest attempt to study the effect of metals on human body was done by Paracelsus, who made the beginning to assess the biocompatibility in the 16th century itself. With the advent of publications of scientific data public new the studies made in this direction. In 1685 the first work in dentistry was published. Pierre Fauchard published Le Chirugien Dentiste in 1728 . John Hunter wrote the natural history of human teeth in 1771 and established dentistry as a separate branch of Medicine. In 179[illegible] John Greenwood developed a foot powered dental drill and fabricated complete denture to George Washington in bone and ivory, which was considered bio-acceptable. 1820-1870 ,the 50 years poured out new ideas on dental materials as a result of organisation of dental education and communication in dentistry. The dental journal emerged in 1840 as American journal of dental science. Such development which took place in materials, of Vulcanite, Porcelain, during that time stimulated dentists to perform clinical and scientific research on new improved materials.

New materials such as celluloid , gutta percha , aluminium and iridium were finding use in dentistry. In 19th century engineering as a science developed application of physics, chemistry and mathematics in the testing of dental materials. In 1861 John Tomes (England) was measuring shrinkage in dental amalgam, Fletcher measured marginal leakage around filling by using dyes, Kirby (1871-1874) used micrometer devices to measure dimensional changes in Amalgam. Dr. Foster Flagg (Philadelphia) evaluated clinical performance of silver amalgam. And 1895 G.V. Black reported the composition of dental amalgam to its physical properties and clinical performance. There was not a phase untouched by Dr. Greene Vardiman Black and his text book on operative dentistry had an enormous influence on the precept and practice which are even followed today.

Pirece (1879) introduced zinc oxide, phosphoric acid and it superseded oxy chloride and oxy sulphate cements because of lesser irritation to pulp and greater durability. Around the same time Dr. Pierce and Dr. J. Foster Flagg originated zinc oxide eugenol cement which is still popular for its obtundent effect. They also acted as luting cement in addition to temporarys. In 1897 Dr. Philbroke of Iwoa demonstrated lost wax for cast gold fillings, but got patented and published by Dr. C .H. Taggart in 1907 using pressure method. An aesthetic material, silicate cement was developed by Thomas Fletcher (England) in 1873 which was improved by Steenbock in 1904. Wells 1883 introduced Nitrous oxide and ether which was used by Morton for painless dental procedures. Kornelis Van Sollingen (1690) remarked penetration of moisture is reduced only with mastic and metallic substances on teeth. G.V.Black recognised that films of contaminant left coating the cavity forming a seal. "Alcohol and Acids will enter where water fails" - such experience with the chemico bacterial theory of dental decay was put forward by W.D. Miller which led Black to advocate scientific cavity preparation to avoid reccurrent marginal leakage and decay. Black also recognised "Galvanic action" due to the use of dissimilar metals and that they should not be 'commingled in the back teeth".

TREND OF BIOLOGICAL TESTING :

Newer materials like acrylic resins generated necessary interest in clinical manifestations of tissue reactions such as acrylic allergy due to the dentures and pulpal reactions to the acrylic fillings. The consequence of physical deficiencies such as setting shrinkage, thermal expansion and corrosion due to marginal leakage, recurrent dentinal caries became apparent. Later in 1950 a trend towards emphasis on biological responses to dental materials was understood by Paffenbarger, Ryge and, they made it obligatory for the denture material researchers to acknowledge and include the biological and clinical aspects. Each year saw development of many more newer dental materials and increasing concern was being expressed to the effect of the material or technique on the soft tissue, and especially dental pulp. In 1960 the need was expanded to have a co-ordinated biological and clinical testing of materials in addition to the measurement of physical and mechanical properties and became accepted as an essential part of the evaluation. Further this investigation was made mandatory by 1970. Earlier materials used in dentistry were mostly from natural sources and they created fewer problems. But as the treatment procedures have become more sophisticated in restorative and preventive techniques, the lack of protection for the patients and the operator and his or her assistants against short term effects of new materials have become more and more evident. Many Governments have intervened and various legislations have been formulated to regulate sale or use of the materials, and to have a monitoring agency. Study of both standardisation and methods of in vitro testing has indicated roots for further progress. They are correlated with in-vivo situations, for better understanding.

EVALUATION OF BIOCOMPATIBILITY CHARACTERISTICS OF DENTAL MATERIALS:

Dental materials are frequently required to fulfill aesthetic as well as functional, preventive or therapeutic purposes and consequently their characterisation is very complex. As there is less information available on the biological properties than physiochemical characteristics, the lacunae is still present to reach an ideal state of knowledge on these dental materials. Placement of dental materials in or on the tissues initiates a two way interaction. The effect of the tissue on the material has to be assessed by the solubility disintegration, corrosion and others. The physiological, pathological, psychological effect of the material on the tissue can also be obvious, but sometimes may be be overlooked as minor. The reaction may be local, remote or may be systemic. Further they may be short term. long term or repetitive , causing sensitivity or allergic manifestations.

1. ***Composition Effects:***

   Zn oxide + Eugenol is very widely used without any control on its purity of ingredients.

   Certain manufacturers have inadvertently used beryllium silicate in silicate cement, which is cytotoxic.

2. ***Physical effects :***

   Amalgam overhangs, composite resins surfaces, subgingival positioning of restorative materials and unsuitable crown morphology can cause mucosal irritation which may arise from preferential growth of organisms. Candida growth on silicon relining materials of artificial dentures was also widely noticed. Certain solid implants may give rise to tumor formations. Interfacial leakage may lead to marginal breakdown and bacterial penetrations.

3. ***Chemical effects :***

I. Short term irritation on the pulp by certain intermediary restorative materials, may lead to necrosis and abscess formation in the long run.

II. Certain materials may decompose and break down, causing leaching of ingredients (cyanoacrylates tissue adhesives).

III. Certain materials result in contact dermatitis or stomatitis due to constant exposure to an agent from the material (nickel, cobalt, copper in gold, polymerization activators, orthodontic elastics.)

4. ***Galvanic phenomenon :***

Electrochemical effects are a special form of chemical activity, since there may be a tissue response due to the flow of current as well as chemical effects of released ions. Corrosion may arise from dissimilar metals in contact, heterogenicity of composition in an alloy or concentration cell conditions. These conditions are more severe when metals or alloys are partly or completely buried in the tissues, as in implants. Cobalt chromium alloys show corrosion with disintegration of elements throughout the body and similar local concentrations of titanium ions. Silver endoposts / points show corrosion in-vivo. Tissue reactions may arise around the base metal bridges and cause formation of lichen planus in humans which have attributed to galvanic action.

5. ***Tumerogenic effects :***

Formation of neoplasm may arise only in special combination of circumstances. Long term exposure to continuing small amounts of chemically carcinogenic agents such as certain aromatic amines, or metals (Ni,Co) may result in tumor formation with an apparent induction period of 12- 25 years in humans. It is also accepted that a physical oncogenic mechanism can exist in relation to implants, which is related to the size and shape of the material. Extremely fine fibers (less than 0.05 micron diameter and 8 micron length) such as several asbestos can enter the cells giving rise to the tumor formation . On the other hand large implants, particularly plates more than 1 cm area may result in elaboration of fibrous tissue capsule, which in turn may produce neoplastic changes; (Oppenheimer effect). The factors are not well understood , but may be related to attachment of tissues to the implant and thickness and vascularity of the fibrous capsules. The induction period may be long and may be variable over a period of time.

6. ***Microbiological consideration :***

This aspect is usually ignored. Bacterial contamination is known to be affected by contamination of dental materials , such as alginate materials, pumice polishing paste, which cause dissemination of hepatitis. Bacterial aerosols can be produced during various dental procedures . Periodontal packs can allow growth of specific organisms at the wound site. The surface of polymers may facilitate the growth of micro-organisms which in turn may degrade the material. There is limited information indicating that certain bacteriae can metabolise some polymers or monomers as a carbon source. There is a demonstrated evidence of microspaces between the tooth and resin surfaces which can harbour bacteriae and allow proliferation. The present day composite resins and sealants may have some limited antibacterial action, compared to older acrylic resins (J Dent Res 57 : 171 :1978 Ostavik D and Heusten- Patterson). The characteristics of materials such as setting shrinkage, swelling due to water sorption, and the chemical characteristic of resins, may influence its tissue reaction in facilitating or **maximizing** the presence of bacteria at the interface of enamel and dentine to initiate caries.

Radiation Effects:

There are several radiations associated with dental materials or devices which may have untoward effects. Two major areas related to dental materials are ultra-violet sources and fluorescent agents in restorative materials. Ultra violet radiation is used in three areas :

- To detect plaque with fluorescent dyes.
- Reveal early carious lesion and emphasize plaque with U V

photography .

- Polymerize composite resin materials and sealants in conjunction with UV activators.

UV radiation can result in damage to the skin, including erythema, sunburns, aging, tumors, damage to the eyes (Photokeratitis). UV wavelengths below 320nm appear to cause most pronounced effects although intensity, duration of exposure, site and susceptibility of the individual are involved. Some may be photosensitive, or made so by the use of certain chemicals like soaps, cosmetics and medicines. Concern has been expressed that excessive exposure to UV by dental procedures might be hazardous to the operator as well as the patient. Guidelines have been issued for the use of UV light and it is advisable to avoid excessive and prolonged exposures.

8. ***Fluorescent Pigments:***

For effective esthetic results certain fluorescent pigments are incorporated in many materials. For many years, compounds containing Uranium and Cerium were employed in the manufacture of ceramic teeth. There are regulations governing the use of Uranium to a very limited extent(0.1% by wt in Germany & 0.05% by wt in the US), and in dental porcelain 0.03% by wt which is a reduction by 40% from the previous levels used. The hazard to our health by the radioactivity of dental porcelain is a debatable issue. The view expressed is that there is negligible danger to the patients but a possible risk to the ceramists. The use of radioactive materials have been discontinued.

CLINICAL OBSERVATIONS:

There may seem to be many possibilities, but little reported evidence of problems in humans compared to the toxicity data derived from animal tests. It is also likely that many clinical toxicological reports are not reported or are overlooked or neglected. In some, they are within the limits of tolerance which may be accepted as routine. Several problems arise with temporary crown & bridge materials. The systemic effect from lead containing alginates through powder inhalation was found to occur among dental assistants (Mjor .Scand.J.Dent Res. 82:401:1974). Mercury pollution and subsequent absorption by dental personnel does occur and it may be minimized by appropriate precautions. Reactions to non precious casting alloys is also observed. Root fractures involving the usage of root canal pins or posts may be associated with corrosion. Hypersensitivity to cobalt and nickel has been reported. Cadmium is present in gold solders (Scand.J.Dent.Res. 85:623:1977. Bergman et al) and in soft metal crowns used in paedodontics. Hazards from asbestos may arise in clinics and dental laboratories. Incidence of mercury sensitivity and type B hepatitis exposure among dental students are on the rise. (J.Am.Dent.Assoc.92:104:1976 White and Brandt and J.Oral Med. 34:33:1979. Gsebal & Gitmick). Many clinicians often lack awareness of these problems, partly due to ignorance of the precise nature of the materials which are being manipulated and placed in the mouth. Appropriate scheme of biocompatibility testing is to be done, and three levels of testing carried out for the evaluation of dental materials.

Level 1: Series of pre-clinical tests in animals and in-vitro studies. These tests can be used as a screening phase but should be followed with more detailed investigations.

Level 2: "In use" tests in animals at the sites where the materials have to be used. The test is similar and duplicated as much as possible as used in humans.

Level 3: Clinical trials in humans, after the data has been sufficiently screened in the first two levels.

TEST METHODS :

1. ***Biological tests:*** Dental materials are classified into five types

   Type I: Materials contacting the body other than the oral cavity through handling, accidental ingestion and inhalation.

   Type II: Materials contacting the mucous membranes and other soft tissues within the oral cavity.

Type III: Materials that might affect health or vitality of the dental pulp or adjacent soft tissues.

Type IV: Root canal filling materials.

Type V: Materials that might affect the health of the hard tissues of the teeth.

The tests are applied to these classes of materials and are selected to the site of application. They are classified into three levels as mentioned in the :

FDI Classification of Biological tests:

Initial Tests:

1. Oral Test
2. Intra peritoneal test (IP test)
3. Inhalation test
4. Haemolysis test
5. Ame's test
6. Style's test
7. Dominant lethal test
8. Cytotoxicity test

Secondary tests: (These tests are related to local tissue toxicity)

1. Subcutaneous implantation test
2. Bone implantation test
3. Sterilization test
4. Oral mucous membrane irritation test

Usage tests: (In vivo- which precede clinical trial in animals- first in Primates and then in humans)

1. Pulp & Dentin test for restorative materials
2. Pulp capping and pulpotomy material test
3. Endodontic material test
4. Endosseous implant material test

Oral test and Intraperitoneal test are essential to determine any acute systemic toxicity of any material tested by the oral and intraperitoneal route. These values are gathered in rats or rabbits and they provide reliable guidance as to whether the material is of high, moderate or low toxicity. Toxicity due to aerosol and gaseous materials are determined by inhalation. Haemolysis test using rabbits blood provide another irritational index. A more sensitive test is that for cytotoxicity. The test material (manipulated as suggested by manufacturers) is observed on cell growth rate or cell lysis in a culture medium in comparison to positive or negative controls. Out of many methods tried by various workers, Spangberg tried a 4 hour and 24 hour observation data of radio-isotope labeled Chromium from lysed cells. These methods are sensitive but may not correlate to the same course of events in higher organisms and especially with regard to long term effects. Pulpal reaction tests in restorative materials can be correlated with these studies but the other tests like cell culture test, implantation and clinical usage tests may give varying results on comparison. In-vitro tests alone cannot be used as a reliable screening test (Bergman. Oral Sci review 10:75:1977). Browne and Tyas have discussed the developments of improved in-vitro tests (Journal of Oral Rehab. 6:365:1979). Two in-vitro tests for mutagenicity are proposed by Ames and Styles.

Ame's test: Utilizes Salmonella typhimurium which do not grow on media and do not contain Histidine. If these bacteria are treated with a mutagen sooner or later there will be a mutation back to the normal state and growth on a histidine-free medium will occur. Thus an index of mutagenic potential of a given chemical can be obtained- if it indicates a high frequency of reserve mutation it will have a high probability of being mutagenic to mammalian species.

Style's test: Is the best known alternative test. "A cell transformation test" signals a potential carcinogen by conversion of normal cultured fibroblast cells from a baby hamster kidney into a quasicancerous state. This transformation has the advantage of using mammalian cells giving a closer resemblance to the whole animal. Both these tests are satisfactory but they do produce a small percentage of false negatives and false positives. Ames claims superiority in his test as it has a strong relationship between mutagenic potential of the test to the carcinogenic potential in animals. Many more tests are necessary to confirm the mutagenicity of the material or the chemical. Dominant lethal test is suggested involving assessment of the injected mutagenic agent on fertility of mice.

Implanting of specimens in animals may give better indications. Selected strains of test animals (rats, mice, hamsters.) give desirable results and the test may last upto two years. Implantation is done subcutaneously and some control group is also retained for comparisons. Constant monitoring for any tissue variation is done. After sacrificing the animal a recommended WHO protocol is observed. An alternative, "local toxicity" is followed in dental materials. They are used for screening purpose. Implantation in soft tissues of rats, mice and guinea pigs as pellets in polyethylene or teflon tubes through surgical incision or rods through intramuscular injection using a trochar. However the use of the tubes are more suitable for the unset and soft materials. The observation periods were 7,30 and 90 days and some studies are done at a less time scale of 2 & 12 days.

Soft tissue area in animals are studied for certain materials used in gums as comparison and materials used as endodontic restorations of bone implants are compared after implantation in bone in animals.

Sensitization test: It is done in Guinea pigs (Magnuson & Kligman) as a two stage induction period. A challenge dose of test material is applied to the skin. After twenty four hours, sensitization rating of redness and swelling is recorded. Many studies are done in this manner for dental materials. Oral mucous membrane is the ideal area for the above test. After the application, the site is observed at one hour and twenty four hours gap and colour changes are recorded. A biopsy is made at the end of twenty four hours. These studies are also made in Hamster cheek or retained on buccal mucosa.

Many acrylic filling materials are tried on rhesus monkeys or baboons where a sterile exposure of pulp is made with a bur and the material used for test capping . The comparison is made with known materials, Calcium hydroxide and saline as control. Inflammatory response and dentin bridging is determined after 3, 90, and 180 days. Similar use of Endodontic filling materials on animal teeth after rootcanal treatment is observed clinically as well as for 180 days and above. If the material passes local and general screening tests , actual usage may invólve manipulative and over above the inherent response of the material. Physical reactions of materials may superimpose microbiological effects. These are clear evidence that pulpal irritation is caused due to marginal leakage and bacterial penetration. There are many direct effects on the pulp due to reaction and irritation, of material in addition to the indirect causes due to physical properties which may lead to defects allowing subsequent bacterial penetration and irritation. For long term assessment of material itself, implantation within the soft tissues seems to be reliable. Endosseous implantation is essentially tested as 7 mm rods inserted in mandibles of Guinea pigs . Similar rods made of Teflon is used as control and tissue reaction assessed after 4-26 weeks. Other galvanic and bio-mechanical tests are to be done in addition to these.

There are many more tests which are to be used and developed. Auto radiography, measurement of vascular changes by Tracers, Dopler, MRI, Scans, are advocated recently.

Ultimately the final biological test depends on actual use in humans .

2. Physical tests:

Main areas of physical methods for testing .

1. *Manipulation of material-* working time , setting time, consistency, odour, colour, setting shrinkage, coefficient of thermal expansion.
2. *Occlusal function-* Parameters of strength, hardness, abrasion resistance, creep, stiffness, viscoelasticity, tooth abrasion, and dissolution.
3. *Aesthetics-* Property of colour, stability of shade, stability of form, resistance to strain, and other parameters simulated in oral conditions.

Most of the tests of dental research relates to materials and physical test methods, which are often done for investigations. They are correlated to standards as prescribed by ADA,FDI,ISO, and ISI.

3. Clinical trials:

After compliance to many in vitro and in vivo trials, clinical trials can be simulated in primates and human volunteers. The guidelines recommended include explanations of-

1. Formulation of the objects. Or Hypothesis of the study.
2. Record keeping.
3. Personnel and their training.
4. Use of reference standards for reliable study criteria.

FUTURE DEVELOPMENT:

Both biological and physical data are essential to characterise a material before clinical trial. Primary studies are to be conducted in live models such as pigs and dogs which may simulate human tooth size and shapes to a near extend.

Biocompatibility of tooth coloured cements and resins :

The principal aim of conservative dentistry is to preserve as much as healthy tissue as possible to enable the pulp of the tooth to respond successfully to the future episodes of disease or iatrogenic trauma.

Silicate restorative materials:

First formulation of silicate was introduced in 1904 by Paul Steeboch in Germany as Ascherís Artificial Enamel. To-day, Composites enjoy more popularity in dental practice but an ideal restorative is not yet discovered. With the severe reaction over pulp use of silicate cement is reduced , but it can still find a use as a temporary filling for caries susceptible young people. Only with the advancement in research and usage of glass ionomer the utility of silicate has become very selective. Research in the area of silicate cements has developed the newer material ion leachable glasses. Earlier the popularity of silicate depended more on its high compressive strength ,aesthetic properties relative to the tooth and its cariostatic quality due to the slow release of fluoride. With proper care and protection over pulp, silicate cements were widely used and had enjoyed the appreciation of many clinicians .The susceptibility to break down during setting of the cement can be reduced by varnish .

BIOLOGICAL EVALUATION:

Cell culture studies.

Silicate was found cytotoxic after setting and the medium adjacent to the surface was made acidic. (Kawahara et al 1968) Investigations to the mechanism of cytotoxicity led to the conclusion that hydrogen ions with fluoride ions derived from it caused toxicity. One brand of silicate was found to contain beryllium 0.7% and another contained 0.2% which has a known cytotoxic effect.

Implantation studies.

Implanted freshly mixed silicate subdermally in rats have shown severe response with necrosis. Specialised implant studies on muscle of rabbits exhibited enzyme activity of silicate cements similar to methyl methacrylate and zinc phosphate cements.

Pulp reaction studies:

Many workers claimed that Silicate cements placed without a lining caused significant pulpal inflammation in humans (Manley, Zander, Seelig, Stanley, Brannstrom, Hansen, Quist). A significant inflammatory reaction of the pulp was also noticed. Barker found a mild reaction with thinning of odontoblastic layer and some round cell reactions. In fact he also reported some secondary dentin formation. There is a consensus of opinion from many pulp studies, that the reaction in the pulp to unlined silicates is universally proportional to the remaining dentin in the cavity. The severity of the reaction to the pulp in the case of unlined silicate fillings has also found to increase with time. Rao stated that the severity of the response to the unlined cement fillings is more acute in the initial 4 weeks and reduced by 12 weeks time. Pulp protection can be effected by selective application of varnish and calcium hydroxide bases.

Gingival tissue response:

Gingival response to silicate fillings is similar to any other filling material such as amalgam and resin and is related to poor oral hygiene, where plaque accumulates with increased production of acids .

Acid theory and pulpal response:

Acid theory states that the production of initial pH of 2 after mixing of silicate cement, gradually rose to 3.9 after 24 hours. It is more acidic than zinc phosphate cements. They also found that 5.72% of acid incorporated in the silicate may be available for diffusion. The acid reactions caused red cell aggregations and thrombolysis with or without antigen antibody reaction. Roydhouse, suggested the acidity is buffered by tissue fluids but the antigen affected the pulp causing a reaction.

Bacterial theory of pulpal damage:

Bacterial layer has been shown to be present under fillings to about 5-20microns. The presence of bacterial toxins was suggested to be the irritant factor. It has also been shown that bacteria can also survive in the presence of silicates even though it has bactericidal properties.

GLASS IONOMER CEMENTS:

This cement is based on the hardening reaction between ion leachable aluminosilicate glass and aqueous solution of polymers and copolymers of acrylic acid. Developed in 1972 to combine silicate and polycarboxylate cements, they are composite materials with embedded glass particles with high abrasion resistance and have an effective bond between filler and matrix due to a chemical reaction. The glass ionomer can adhere to enamel, dentin, stainless steel, tin, tin oxide plated platinum and gold. They are not adherent to porcelain and pure forms of gold and platinum. When Glass ionomer cements were introduced the pulp response was classified as bland, safe, moderate and less irritating to the earlier tooth coloured materials. The blandness of glass ionomer cements was attributed to the absence of strong acids, and monomers.

Polyacrylic acid and related polyacids are much weaker than phosphoric acid and poses much higher molecular weight that may limit diffusion through the dentinal tubules into the pulp. The other acids were added to modify the polyacrylic acid and to increase the reactivity with the glass particles. Certain water setting formulations in glass powder was blended with polyacrylic powder and the mix was made with the addition of water. The elimination of viscous poly acid solution yielded a satisfactory mix.

Biological evaluation

Irritation of pulp due to poly acrylic acid is less because:

a. It is a weak acid.

b. It is strongly bound to the area of poly anion chain by electrostatic forces.

c. Its diffusion down the dentinal tubules is restricted due to high molecular weight as polymer and entangled by Polymeric chain.

Cell culture studies.

In experiments with prolonged cell contact time with specimens which had set for twenty four hours the material appeared to be non toxic. This is in contrast with same technique in experiments with conventional silicate cements which appeared to have a lasting toxic effect. Comparing the cytotoxicity of poly carboxylates and glass ionomers , marked cytotoxic reaction was noted with polycarboxylate and this may be due to the presence of zinc in the powder and the differences in setting reaction.

Smith and Ruse (1986) compared initial acidity of glass ionomer with Zn polycarboxylate and Zn phosphate cements and formed a general risk of pH for all cements during the first 15 minutes. But the initial reaction of glass ionomer was slow leaving an acidic pH of 2.0 at 5 minutes and 3.0 at 10 minutes time.

Stanley and Pameijer (1984) found pulp abscess and hemorrhage when the remaining dentine thickness was less than 0.5 mm. Ideally a base of calcium hydroxide under glass ionomer cement should be ideal and particularly when the remaining dentine thickness is 1mm or less.

Pulpal Studies.

Mild pulp reaction was noted in a week's time after application on tooth. Earlier method of conditioning with "citric acid" was found to cause more pulpal irritation than when not conditioned.

Clinical trials.

Class V cavity restored with glass ionomer cement did not present any gingival reaction. Eventhough the cavity were not lined relief from sensitivity was claimed. The glass ionomer with its encouraging clinical results may develop into a future tooth coloured material of choice.

COMPOSITE RESINS.

Bio compatibility

All acrylic restorative materials inclusive of composites are toxic to the pulp as indicated by Stanley et al. Stanley , Langerland and Suraẹz have recommended the use of a bulk liner under the composite restorations. Cytotoxicity procedures proposed by Spanburg are recommended for biological evaluation of dental materials.They are tested for cytotoxicity, Haemolysis, Ame's Test ,Styles Test for all cell transformation, pulp irritation usage test. The ingredients and their combinations are stûdied by animal experiments. Class V cavities are made in monkey teeth for studying the effect of BIS-GMA ,Triethylene glycol dimethacrylate, a barium glass, methyl ether of hydroquinone, benzyl peroxide, p-tolyl diethanolamine, benzoin methyl ether. All the studies pointed out the apparent cause of the pulpal involvements in that there is an attempt to separate chemical material factors from effects due to marginal leakage and bacterial invasion.

Marginal leakage and bacterial invasion .

Zander(1950) reported resins are not directly responsible for pulp irritation but was due to microleakage which allowed dentine to be exposed to oral environment. Brannstrom reported that composite shrink from the cavity walls on setting. On comparison of composites with silicate and non composite resins pulpal response was very similar in quantity and quality. The amount of remaining dentin was the factor for variations of effect. Bacterial invasion was also noticed under all the restorations after a period of time. Nondenvall and Brannstrom studied whether the acid etching would prevent growth of bacterial colonies. Neither the acid treatment nor the enamel bond resin caused any significant damage to the pulp.

Acid etch technique.

Many studies done on test animals indicated acid etching appeared to make dentine more permeable to the deleterious agent of composite resin.

Retif used 50% Phosphoric acid on monkey teeth for 1 minute and filled the cavities. They concluded 50% phosphoric acid produced a more severe pulpal response than control teeth and suggested use of protective liner to cover the exposed dentin before etching adjacent enamel.

UNFILLED AND FILLED RESINS.

Effect on pulp.

Both resulted irritation to the dental pulp. A neutral base ($Ca(OH)2$)has been recommended as a protective layer.

Effect on Gingiva.

Gingival tissues adjacent to restorations with sub gingival margins developed marginal gingivitis. Plaque also formed very easily. This may be due to relatively large fillers in filled resins.

RESIN BONDED COMPOSITE CEMENTS (DUAL CURE)

Relatively low viscosity of resin cements reduces the possibility of less voids and proper restorative seating with less pressure. Due to the bonding potential the resin based cements are increasing the fracture resistance of all ceramic crowns. 1992, Stanley Pameijer compared pulp response of dual cured resin based cements to light cured and chemically cured resins. Light curing adequately done is safer and the chemically cured resins exceeded the accepted level of biocompatibility. More solution and less powder increased the possibility of diffusion within dentine. Increase in conditioning time and hydraulic pressure increases severity of pulp responses.

CONDITIONING (ACID ETCHING AGENTS):

Both composites and glass ionomer use conditioning or etching. The conditioning or etching are of high acid concentration, when applied to extended intervals remove the layer and dentinal plugs, funnel the tubular orifices , denature the exposed collagen fibers and increase the potential for severe pulp responses.

The conditioning of freshly cut dentine allows removal of smear layer and causes ingress of bacteria and outward flow of dentinal fluid, possibly contributing to the formation of a bio film interfering with adhesion - Brannstorm (1981). So many of them recommend retaining the smear layer. Further studies made a suggestion that conditioning should be limited to 15 secs and not to 2 mins. Mount (1990) also suggested 5 secs for conditioning as a safer method.

Bavlar et all (1982) introduced a mordenting solution (acidified ferric oxalate replaced later by aluminium oxalate) which appears to dissolve the existing smear layer and leave a uniform artificial altered smear layer which gave a better control of the pulp reaction. Bowen and Blosser (1988) suggested a solution of aluminium nitrate 2.5 %, oxalic acid and 1.5 %, 2.4 % nitric acid and 5 % N-phenyl glycine used on the surface for 60 secs were effective as conditioning agents (not using ferric and aluminium oxalate). These surface modifications on dentine should limit to 10 microns and not deeper.

BONDING AGENTS :

No significant pulp response was noticeable to any bonding agents and they do not appear to be toxic. (1991) Stanley Pameijer evaluated the PRISMA universal bond -2 a two component no-mix system composed of dentine primer and adhesive.

Primer - 30 % Hydroxyethyl methacrylate (HEMA)

- 64% ethanol &
- PENTA (Di penta - aerythritol penta acrylate phosphoric acid) 6% an adhesive
- Acid ester 6%.

This did not remove smear layer and was hydroxyphilic. It showed increased micromechnical bonding and no chemical reaction to dentine. The Primer was used after etching the surface for 60 secs with 37 % phosphoric acid. Very low to average inflammatory response was noted. Pulp changes may vary due to age changes in the teeth.

Although a wide spectrum of materials, devices exists in diverse surgical disciplines as opthalmology, cardiology , neurology, orthopedics, and dentistry they all have one thing in common. They must have intimate contact with human tissues , providing real, classical physical interface. The term bio compatibility has come into existance with referance to the study of interaction of various materials with human tissues.

"Absolute bio compatibility may be regarded as utopia,while in more realistic way we have to consider the degree of bio compatibility that we find in practice" . D. Williams.

ELASTOMERIC SILICONE IMPRESSION MATERIALS AND IMPRESSION PROCEDURES

Solomon E.G.R.

Introduction

Silicone elastomers are composed of organic polymethylsiloxanes derived from silicates, which enclose oxygen atoms and organic compounds. Commercially two types of silicone impression materials are available for various types of impressions encountered in clinical practice. Condensation reaction silicones consists of polymethylsiloxane as the basic polymer and accelerators which are esters of silicic acid. The addition reaction silicones consists of polymethylvinylsiloxane and polymethylhydrogen siloxane as the basic polymer. The chemical reaction of these two materials are different from the other. In condensation reaction silicone, no change in the basic structure takes place during setting. The chemical reaction is accompanied by volatilisation, whereas in addition reaction silicone a total transformation takes place. The final product is different after the completion of setting reaction. The chemical reaction does not produce loss of weight nor decrease in volume of the set elastomer. Condensation reaction and additional reaction silicones should not be mixed as they are chemically incompatible.

Presently cross-linking addition silicones which offer good thixotrophic properties with excellent precision and dimensional stability even if the impression is stored for several days are available.

Physical Characteristics of Elastomers - Clinical Importance :

1. Elongation (Extensibility) : It is the extension of the material up to its rupture or tearing. It is a measure of the ability of material to resist elongation during removal of the impression (Eg.) 100%

means that the elastomer has the ability to double its original length before it tears.

2. Tensile Strength : It is the load required to reach breaking point (Eg.) kg/cm^2 means that the breaking occurs when a force equal to this value is applied.

3. Module of Elasticity : "Module E" at 50%. It is the strength necessary to obtain 50% elongation, it indicates the rigidity of the elastomer.

4. Elasticity and Elastic Limits : Ability to recover to initial form after constraints are removed. Limits of elasticity indicates the force beyond which a permanent deformation takes place. It indicates the elastic capacity of elastomers and beyond its limits produce permanent elastic deformation. This is a measure of the adaptability of silicone impressions during its removal from undercut areas.

5. Elastic Deformation : When a force acts on the impression, it modifies its shape, and if it recovers its form after the elimination of force, it is known to have elastic deformation (Eg.). 6% elastic deformation, it means that the material can reach a maximum elongation of 6%, beyond this point it is not able to recover to its oringal shape.

6. Elastic Recovery : The capability of the material to recover after the force is withdrawn. It is elastic defomation of a sample elongated by 50% in 10 minutes duration.

7. Permanent Deformation : When constraints are removed it does not recover to its oringal shape.

(Eg.) 2% permanent deformation means, that the elastomer showed a variation of 2% after removal of constraints.

8. Tear Resistance : The force required to reach the tear point of the elastomer. 1.00 kg/cm^2 means that a strength of 1.00 kg is necessary to break a sample with a cross section of 1 cm^2.

9. Hardness : Resistance to penetration, measured with a hardness tester. It is tested with shore needles and expressed as 30 degree shore A, 70 degree shore A etc.

10. Dimensional Stability : Linear change of elastomer sample length after setting is complete. It is related to time.

11. Cold Flow : It is the deformation of the material by its own weight. Material with low viscosity exhibit cold flow greater than high viscous materials. (Eg.) Cold flow. 07 means that under constant force (force more than its force of gravity) after 1 hr the height of the sample is reduced 0.07 times as compared to its orignal value.

12. Consistency : The elastomer mix is compressed with a definite force between two slabs. The dispersal of the material indicates the consistency of the elastomer.

13. Viscosity : It is the degree of internal friction of particles contained under displacement. It significantly affects the dispersability, surface reproduction details and surface tension. It is measured by viscosimeters and value expressed in centipose units. (Eg.) Brookefield. Heavy bodied elastomers have greater viscosity than medium and high bodies.

(Eg.)	Heavy Body	4,50,000 cps
	Light Body	45,000 cps

14. Setting Curve : Expresses the ratio between increase in viscosity of elastomer with the measure of time.

15. Surface Tension : It is the attraction power of all materials, caused by the difference of attractions of atoms by the surface of materials. It is an indicator of the ability of wetting a surface. Wettability can be increased by the use of wetting agents.

16. Deterioration : The loss of efficiency of elastoemer resulting from time factor or due to a particular circumstance such as temperature. It is measure of the ability of a material to keep its performance over a long period of time.

17. Thixotrophy : Ability to support against gravity without slumping. A very important requirement to keep the material around the gingival margins in upper arch,.

IMPRESSION PROCEDURES WITH SILICONES

I. Double Impression Technique - Wash Technique - Reline Technique -

Corrective Impression Technique

First Impression is taken with a high viscous silicone such as putty or heavy bodied silicone. After its setting is complete the impression is removed, trimmed of its undercuts and relined with a light bodied silicone, and a second impression is taken over the primary impression of heavy bodied silicone.

Although the accuracy of impression is good, it exhibits deformation due to the release of compressive forces upon removal of the second impression. It is important that no pressure is exerted during the setting of secondary impression. If pressure is exerted during the setting of the secondary impression, then it results in the incorporation of stress in the elastic primary impression, which is released upon the removal of secondary impression from the mouth, resulting in its distortion. Pressure causes compression and displacement of elastic primary impression, which in turn results in the deformation of the set light bodied elastomer, as the compressed heavy bodied elastomer springs back to its normal position after the tray is removed from the mouth.

To minimise the error, pressure is maintained only for a few seconds to permit the light bodied material to flow around the preparation, subsequently the tray is held in neutral position without any pressure till the material sets.

II. Modified Double Impression Technique

The procedure of recording impression is almost similar to that of double impression technique. An initial primary impression of the dental arch is taken in heavy bodied or putty material before the abutment preparation is done. After the completion of tooth preparation, this primary impression is used as a custom tray and a secondary corrective lining impression is taken with light bodied silicone. The pressure treatment of secondary impression is important. The same procedure as in case of double impression technique is meticulously followed.

III. Double Mix Technique - Two Phase Impression

It is a method of recording impression simultaneously with two different viscosities of silicone elastomers. Initially a low viscosity light bodied silicone is injected around the gingival margins and preparations or inlay cavity with a syringe. An impression is then taken with either a high viscosity heavy bodied or putty material which forces the light bodied silicone to flow around the tooth preparation. Pressure is maintained till both the materials set. Since the light and heavy bodied silicone set simultaneously there is no incorporation of stress or strain in the impression as it happens with double impression technqiue. However in this technique subgingival penetration of impression material is limited, becuase of low compression. Therefore sharp margins are not always reproduced. Further the heavy bodied material in the tray can displace the light bodied material on the tooth preparation in a few areas.

IV. Monophase or Single Impression Technique :

One of the simplest, easiest and quickest method to record impression for inlays and abutment tooth preparations. Impression is recorded with one impression material, in contrast to double impression and double mix techniques, where two different viscosities are used.

Polyether is the ideal material for monophase impression. Polyether has better thixotrophic property than silicones. However the recently introduced cross-linking addition silicones claim good thixotrophism. This technique requires the preparation of custom tray with spacer. Intially the cavity preparation or the gingival margin and preparation surface as the case may be is injected with a medium bodied silicone or polyether elastomer. The custom tray is then loaded with the same mix of elastomer and it is seated over the dental arch and impression is recorded under moderate pressure till the elastomer sets.

Summary : Silicone elastomers permit several consistencies to be achieved. It is available in four consistencies; a thin easy flowing light bodied, a more viscous creamy medium bodied and a highly viscous heavy bodied. Besides these, it is also possible to have silicone in the form of kneadable putty consistency. All these can be used either individually or in combination with each other. Silicone elastomer is also used as a substitute for low fusing compound with a copper band. It gives good surface details and gingival reproduction when used as a single impression or when light and heavy bodied/putty are combined together in one impression.

ROOT-END FILLING MATERIALS IN SURGICAL ENDODONTICS

Subba Rao C.V.

INTRODUCTION :

The Prime objective of Root Canal therapy is to achieve a perfect hermetic seal of the apical foramen. When non-surgical attempts proved unsuccessful or contra-indicated, surgical endodontic therapy followed by retrofilling is the treatment of choice. With the advent of modern materials and technology, one can achieve high degree of success in endodontic therapy.

According to Gartner and Dorn,[8] an ideal material to seal the root-end cavities should prevent leakage of microorganisms and their by-products into periapical tissues. It should also be non-toxic, non-carcinogenic and biocompatible with host tissues. In addition, it should be insoluble in tissue fluids and dimensionally stable. Further, the presence of moisture should not affect their sealing ability. It should be easy to manipulate, fast-setting and radiopaque.

Various materials have been tried as retrofilling materials namely Gutta-Percha, Silver Amalgam, Polycarboxylate cement, Zinc Phosphate cement, Zinc-Oxide eugenol paste, IRM, EBA cement, Cavit, Glass Ionomers, Composite resins and other materials such as Gold Foil, Silver points, Cyanoacrylates, Poly HEMA and Hydron, Diaket root canal sealer, Titanium screws and Teflon. Recently, Titanium inlay with Super EBA cement as a sealer was tried as a new root-end filling material.[9,31]

AMALGAM :

Amalgam has been used as a retrofilling material for the past 5 decades. It is most popular due to easy manipulation, good radiopacity, non-solubility in tissue fluids. As the amalgam restoration ages marginal adaptability and sealing was improved due to formation of corrosion products. It has been demonstrated experimentally that amalgam corrodes and it releases potential toxic ions and chemicals. Tissue irritation may exist due to breakdown products of amalgam. It has been suggested by Omnell. KA [16] that zinc free amalgam was preferred as retrofilling material. He further claimed that electrolysis occurs around zinc containing alloys and this precipitates zinc carbonate into the tissues which retards healing of periapical tissues.

The sealing ability of amalgam depends upon the depth of retrograde cavity. It was found that 3 mm of amalgam retrofill significantly reduce apical leakage compared to 1 mm and 2 mm retrofillings according to Mattison. GD et al (1985).[13]

In case of high copper, zinc-free amalgam there is a less susceptibility to corrosion, less creep value, high strength and no obvious delayed expansion in clinical conditions.[11]

Immediately after restoration with amalgam, shrinkage and setting expansion of 10µm/cm occur which creates space between amalgam and canal wall due to slow setting of the material. The formation of microspace may result in poor adaptation of amalgam which has been confirmed by SEM studies.[14]

In clinical situations, the above mentioned microleakage can be overcome by the application of cavity varnish, which will reduce the microleakage significantly. Due to its disadvantages such as release of mercury and tin ions, corrosion, amalgam tatoo, delayed expansion, initial marginal leakage and possiblity of scattering at periapical region. Search for newer materials were undertaken by many investigators.

GUTTA PERCHA :

Gutta percha as a retrofilling material was used in conjunction with chloropercha. Thermoplasticized form was tried so that the retrofilling material has been well adapted to cavity walls. The orthograde gutta percha root canal obturation that is frequently associated with apical surgery is burnished after apicoectomy with either a hot or cold burnisher. [10]

Abdal. AK, etal studied the apical seal by heat sealed gutta percha and the heat sealed gutta percha reinforced with composite dental resin. They concluded that the reinforced gutta percha provided the most effective seal.

Due to its porous nature, it absorbs moisture from the surrounding periapical tissue and expands intially which is followed by contraction in later stage. This may result in poor marginal adaptation and increased microleakage.

Since amalgam and guttapercha fail to provide ideal apical seal other substances such as zinc oxide eugenol based cements, glass ionomers, composites, etc have been tried as root end filling materials.

REINFORCED ZINC OXIDE AND EUGENOL CEMENTS :

In recent years, reinforced zinc oxide and eugenol cements have become accepted as the non-metallic root-end filling material of choice. Specifically, the materials that have been recommended are IRM and Super EBA cement. These materials were developed in an attempt to increase the strength and reduce the setting time of ZOE cements. IRM is reinforced with polymethylmethacrylate, and SuperEBA cement is reinforced with alumina. Super EBA contains 37.5% eugenol compared to IRM's 99%. The eugenol in IRM, however, is not readily released because of the effect of dispersion of the resin particles. The ingredients of these two materials are as follows:

IRM :

Powder: zinc oxide - 80% : Polymethylmethacrylate - 20%

Liquid : acetic acid-1 % ; eugenol - 99%

Super EBA

Powder: Zinc oxide - 60%; alumina - 34% ; natural resin - 6%

Liquid : Ortho-ethoxy benzoic acid - 62.5%; eugenol - 37.5%

Numerous studies have been reported and have found favourable results in sealing ability, tissue tolerance, and clinical success for both IRM and EBA. EBA generally is considered to provide a superior seal, and several studies [3,4,21] claim that EBA demonstrates virtually no leakage. Leakage studies of IRM have shown both good and poor results depending on how the material is manipulated. Although, all materials are cytotoxic to some degree, both IRM and EBA seem to be well tolerated by tissues in studies done to date.[10]

Few clinical studies have been done to evaluate these materials in vivo. Amalgam has been shown in numerous studies to average 70% to 75% success rate. In a retrospective study of 488 cases done in two distinct geographic locations over a 10 year period, Dorn and Gartner reported identical 75% success rates for amalgam, whereas IRM and Super EBA showed success rates of 91% and 94% respectively. The results were statistically significant and indicate that the use of IRM or Super EBA as root-end filling materials appears favourable.[8]

The sealing ability of IRM with the addition of 10-20% of hydroxyapatite (HAP) was studied by using a confocal optical microscope with a fluorescent dye.[17] This was compared with another reinforced zinc oxide eugenol cement (Kalzinol), EBA cement and amalgam. it was concluded that IRM and Super EBA cement showed better sealing ability, However, the addition of 10-20% HAP did not affect the sealing ability of IRM.

Manipulation of the Materials :

EBA cements are reinforced with either aluminium oxide or silicon dioxide. The optimum percentage of aluminium oxide to provide ideal physical properties is 34%. This formulation can be found in Super EBA. Super EBA cement is packaged with a regular set and a fast set powder. The fast set powder is the only one that should be used for surgical procedures.

The Super EBA powder and liquid should be mixed on a glass slab with a metal spatula to a very thick, firm consistency, incorporating as much powder as possible. The material then can be transferred to the apical preparation with a curved Messing gun. This instrument is excellent for producing a dense, bubble-free root-end filling but must be kept meticulously clean. Alternately, a cement paddle or the convex side of a bone curette can be used to place the material into the preparation.

A surgical condensor should be used to compact the material into the preparation, after dipping the condensor in the powder to prevent material from sticking to it. Super EBA adheres well to itself and can be added incrementally as necessary. Any excess material can be removed with bone curettes or periodontal curettes. As a final step, it is very important to burnish the material toward the margins. This step will insure that there are no open margins.[10]

IRM is available as a powder and a liquid or in a pre-measured capsules. Hand mixing is preferable because the capsules tend to produce a wet and sticky mix with an uneven consistency. The powder and liquid should be mixed in a 1:4 (liquid:powder) ratio on a glass slab. Based on in vitro studies, the manufactuer's recommended proportion produces increased leakage and an excessively dry mix.

IRM should be placed into the root-end preparation as a single mass because this material does not adhere well to itself and cannot be added incrementally. Unlike Super EBA, IRM is a dry material and tendes to flake or leave open margins if mishandled. The material should thus be wiped into the preparation in one increment with the convex side of a bone curette or with a cement paddle. After trimming away any excess, the IRM should be burnished towards the margins with a ball burnisher. Do not wipe the IRM with a wet cotton pellet, as this will roughen the surface and might open a margin and therefore increase leakage.

Super EBA and IRM are radiopaque but do not have the same density as amalgam. Radiopacifiers such as barium sulfate or amalgam powder should not be added in an attempt to increase the radiographic density of these materials. This may change their properties, affect their seal, or result in an amalgam tattoo.[10]

TABLE

COMPARISON OF THE PROPERTIES OF SEVERAL MATERIAL

	Material			
Property	**ZOE**	**IRM**	**Super EBA**	**Cavit**
% Eugenol	85-100%	99%	37.5%	none
Released eugenol	50-80%	4%	2%	none
Strength	2000 lbs/in	800 lbs/in	5600 lbs/in	250 lbs/in
Solubility	high (2,5%)	low (<0.1%)	moderate (1%)	very high (10%)
Hardness	low	highest	high	very slow
Sealability	very good	good	excellent	excellent

Cavit :

It is a synthetic, zinc oxide based temporary filling material. It has been used as a retrofilling material primarily due to its ease of application which does not require any manipulation or mixing. It is a hygroscopic material which expands as a result of water absorption during setting. Consequently its adaptation to cavity wall is expected to be good. But possibly a minimum thickness of material is required for optimal seal to be obtained. Since the setting of cavit is enhanced by tissue fluids, in vivo studies it is found to be soluble and quickly disintegrated.[9,10]

The results obtained from the animal experiements showed that the tissue response to IRM, Super EBA and Cavit were similar and mild and is less severe than ZOE and Kalzinol.[19]

ZOE :

ZOE seals well but demonstrates a surface softness and tendency for disintegration. In addition, unreinforced ZOE releases eugenol when the set eugenolate contacts moisture. Eugenol is cytotoxic to connective tissue, reversibly neurotoxic, potentially immunogenic, and damaging to epithelium. In low concentration however, eugenol stimulates fibroblast formation, inhibits prostaglandin synthesis, antimicrobial and provides a sedative effect. Because ZOE provides an excellent seal, an ideal root-end filling material would be a ZOE cement modified to decrease solubility and reduce eugenol release. [10]

ZINC POLYCARBOXYLATE CEMENT :

It consists of zine oxide, magnesium oxide and small amounts of aluminium oxide mixed with water solution of polyacrylic acid. Since it has a property of adhesion to tooth structure by chelating with calcium, it has been considered as a potential retrofilling material. Further it has been noticed that the adherence of polycarboxylate cement to dentin is lesser than the enamel. The bond to dentin is adversely affected by moisture and protein contamination such as contact with blood or saliva. It is hardly soluble in water. Hence it is advantageous as retrofilling material. In a vital tissue, it may partly get absorbed. The applicatlon of this cement is difficult as a result of its viscosity and because of acceleration of its setting reaction in warm environment.[10]

OTHER MATERIALS:

Teflon, Poly HEMA (Hydron), zinc phosphate cement and diaket has been tried as retrofiling materials.

Poly HEMA (Hydron) requires 24 hours to cure, entraps air bubbles, is cytotoxic to tissues and is very difficult to use.

Teflon is very tissue tolerant but seals very poorly in the presence of moisture.

Diaket, a zinc oxide polyketone vinyl resin, has been used by some clinicians. However, it is strongly cytotoxic for the first 24 hours, produces long term chronic inflammation and gives a poor seal in a wet field.[10]

Cyanoacrylates stimulate acute inflammation, demonstrate high monomer release and need more research before they can be advocated.

GOLD FOIL :

There are studies[33, 34] conducted using gold leaves as retrograde filling material and radiographs showed excellent bone healing in apical region. Gold leaf was used in the form of fine and pure gold. The advantages claimed are its malleability, condensability, sealing ability, easy manipulation, homogenous surface due to its cohesivenss, no tarnish or corrosion and no setting time. It can be sterilized by autoclaving or heating or immersion in 70% ethanol.

GLASS IONOMER:

The advantage of using GIC as retrofilling material is its ability to adhere to tooth structure which results in superior seal. Use of conventional GI as retrofilling material was found to be superior than silver amalgam according to many workers. [2,5] However, the setting reaction of glass ionomer cement is adversely affected by hydration and dehydration, both of which are difficult to control clinically. Hence, the suitability of this type of GIC as a retrofilling material is questioned. It has been claimed that the latest generation of GIC's are less affected by mositure and better suited as retrofilling material for clinical use. The other disadvantage of conventional GIC is lack of radiopacity. It is sticky and its application as retrofilling material is difficult. The application is usually facilitated by syringe.

It has been claimed [18;22] that silver reinforced glass ionomer has improved physical properties compared to conventional glass ionomer, such as high packing density, low porosity, ability to bond to dentin chemically, short setting time, radiopacity, no chipping or flaking during finishing process.

In 1980, glass ionomer powder was modified by incorporating Ag-Sn particles. The formulation was called 'Miracle Mix'. The short-coming observed in this combination was that the fillers do not strongly adhere to the matrix. Hence, Ag-Pd was introduced. This Ag-Pd combination generated an oxide film of Pd oxide which is chemically reactive by chelation with polyacrylic acid and this combination was termed as 'Cermets'.

Walls. AWG (1987)[35] reported that high temperature sintering of silver into glass ionomer powder has added radiopacity to the material and rendering the cement as a potential retrofilling material compared to conventional GIC.

The only drawback of this cement is its moisture sensitivity. During surgery, it is difficult to control moisture which may interfere with the bonding of the cement to hard tissues resulting in poor apical seal.

Recently Light cured, resin reinforced GIC has been introduced. Due to its improved physical properties and better apical seal, this material has been tried as a retrofilling material by Chong. BA, et al (1991),.[6] They claimed that the least micro leakage observed in their study may be due to, less moisture sensitivity, less curing shrinkage, deeper penetration of polymers into the dentin surface and presence of HEMA further enchances the affinity between the dentin and cement.

Spectrometric depth profile studies were conducted by Lin.A, et al (1992)[12] and reported that there is ionic movement from light cured glass ionomer into dentin surface to the depth of 1.5 mm and exchange of calcium and phosphate from dentin into the cement to a depth of 1 mm.

It has been observed that the light cured glass ionomer adapts well to one of the walls of the cavity, whereas gaps were observed on the opposite wall. This gap at the interface can be attributed to polymerization contraction. It has been reported that forces of polymerization were greater than the adhesion of the material to the cavity wall.[7]

The polymerization shrinkage can be reduced to some extent by the incremental curing of the material.

COMPOSITE RESIN :

Composites of different types have been tested as retrofilling material. They were used as retrofilling material even before bonding them to dentin became a possibility. [1,2,4] The currently available modality of bonding composite resin to dentin improves their sealing ability which may be advantageous to the application of composite resins as a retrofilling materials. However the efficacy of dentin bonding system for the composite resin is reduced by exposure of the prepared dentin surface to moisture.

Depending on the type of material used, the composite resins, are placed in the retrocavities by a plastic instrument or by a syringe. Light cured composite resin offer the advantage that it has command setting.

Rud. J, et al (1991) tried the gluma bonding agent followed by application of chemically curable composite containing silver for radiopacity. They observed successful results in most cases. The main cause of failure was considered to be due to inadequate hemostasis or root fracture unnoticed during filling.[20]

The sealing ability of four dentin bonding agents - Amalgam bond, Scotch bond multipurpose, Prisma Universal Bond 3, and All Bond 2 was evaluated by Vignaroli. PA, et al (1995)[32] They applied these materials directly to the resected root end without retrograde cavity preparation. Result indicated that all dentin bonding agents significantly reduced apical microleakage compared to control group. Further, they reported that the blood contamination did not affect the sealing ability of the above mentioned dentin bonding agents except All-Bond 2 group.

MINERAL TRIOXIDE AGGREGATE (MTA):

Torabinejad.M, et al (1995)[29,30] used MTA as retrofilling material in vitro. They determined the chemical composition, pH, radiopacity, setting time and compressive strength. The main molecule present in MTA are calcium and phosphorous ions by using X-ray energy dispersive spectrometer in conjunction with SEM. The pH value was assessed with pH meter which showed that MTA has a pH of 10.2 initially and rises to 12.5 three hours after mixing. It was more radiopaque than Super EBA and IRM. It has longest setting time of about 2 hours and 45 minutes, compressive strength of about 40 MPa and very low solubility. It has antibacterial effect on some of the facultative bacteria and no effect on the strict anaerobic bacteria.

LASER:

Laser technology has been tried (CO^2 and Nd : YAG) on the periapical region at the root tip. The effect of Nd : YAG laser on permeability of apical dentin following apicoectomy and retrofilling has been investigated by Stabholz.A(1992).[25] He observed that the application of laser to the root surface changed its surface permeability and reduce the permeability in resected roots.

TITANIUM INLAY:

Sumi.Y, et al (1997)[28] tried titanium inlay with Super EBA cement as a sealer, as a new root end filling material following periradicular surgery. This was combined with ultrasonic root end preparation technique. The post operative observation have shown encouraging results. Titanium was used because of its good biocompatibility. It has excellent corrosion resistance because it forms a protective oxide film on its surface. It has been reported that a physiological seal can be achieved at a root apex by formation of tissue simulating bone, cementum or dentin with materials such as tricalcium phosphate and decalcified allogenic bone graft. They reported that the above materials initiates cementogenesis and osteogenesis at root apex. [15, 23]

EVALUATION OF RETROFILLING MATERIALS :

The evaluation of the suitability of potential retrofilling materials for their intended use has been the purpose of numerous studies. The investigated aspects of the materials are mainly their sealing ability, marginal adaptation, biocompatibility, and their clinical efficacy.

The sealing ability and marginal adaptation of retrofilling materials has been evaluated by many investigators.[9] The following methods have been tried, such as dye penetration method by using indian ink, silver nitrate, aniline dye, methylene blue dye, fluorescent dye, crystal violet dye, radio isotope penetration, bacterial penetration, fluid filtration method, fluorometric analysis, spectrometry and SEM study.

Currently, there are three recommended tests to evaluate the biocompatibility of dental restorative materials. An initial test which provides general toxicity profile of potential materials, secondary tests which evaluate local toxicity and usage tests in which the potential substances are used in the teeth of experimental animals according to clinical protocol.

Cytotoxicity test is one of the most commonly used in vitro tests to measure biocompatibility. It is simple, rapid and inexpensive screening test. The cytotoxicity tests frequently used include agar overlay technique, millipore filter method and radiochromium release test. Invivo subcutaneous and intraosseous implantation techniques in animals are used to evaluate the biocompatibiity.[31]

ANTIBACTERIAL EFFECT :

It has been reported that dental restorative materials such as Ag amalgam, GI cement, resin modified GI, Poly acid modified composite resin (Dyract), fluoride containing composite (Heliomolar), polycarboxylate and dentin bonding agent containing glutaraldehyde which are used as retrofilling materials have antibacterial efficiency.[27]

CONCLUSION :

Retrofilling is a clinically valuable procedure, promoting the prognosis of apical surgery.

The choice of retrofilling material is based on the experimental data. Clinical evaluation and experiments performed invivo are more relevant than studies performed invitro. Animal studies can be considered as a valuable adjunct to the clinical evaluation of retrofilling materials. Silver amalgam is still widely used as a retrofilling material. In some countries, the use of amalgam is prohibited. Hence to select appropriate retrofilling material, further research on newer materials are in progress.

REFERENCES :

1. Abdal.AK, Retief. DH and Jamison.HC: The apical seal via the retrosurgical approach, Oral Surg 54(2) : 213, 1982.

2. Barkhordar.RA, Pelzner.RB and Scark.MM : Use of glass ionomers as retrofilling materials, Oral Surg Oral med Oral Pathol J 67: 734-739... 1989.

3. Beltes.P, Zervas.P, Lambrianidis.T and Molyvdas.I: Invitro study of the sealing ability of four retrograde filling materials, Endod Dent Traumatol 4: 82-84, 1988.

4. Bondra.DL, Hartwell.GR, Mac Pherson.MG and Portell.FR: Leakage invitro with IRM, high copper amalgam and EBA cement as retrofilling materials, J Endod 15(4) : 157-160, 1989.

5. Callis. PD & Santini. A : Tissue response to retrograde root fillings in the ferret canine : A comparison of a glass ionomer cement and gutta percha with sealer. Oral Surg Oral Med Oral Pathol J 64 : 475-479, 1987.

6. Chong. BS, Pitt Ford. TR & Watson. TF : The adaptation and sealing ability of light-cured glass ionomer retrograde root fillings, Int Endod J 24: 223-232, 1991.

7. Chong. BS, Pitt Ford. TR & Watson. TF : Light-cured glass ionomer cement as a retrograde root seal. Int Endod J 26 : 218-224, 1993.

8. Dorn. So & Gartner. AH : Retrograde filling materials - A retrospective success - failure study of amalgam, EBA & IRM, J Endod 16 (8) : 391-393, 1990.

9. Friedman. S : Retrograde approaches in endodontic therapy, Endod Dent Traumatol 7:97-107, 1991.

10. Hovland. EJ : Endodontic, DCNA 36 (2) : Pg 357-378, 1992.

11. Ingle. JI & Langeland.K : Textbook of Endodontics. Chapter - 15: 618-707, Third Edition, 1985.

12. Lin. A, Mcintyre & Davidson. RA : Studies on the adhesion of glass ionomer cements to dentin. J Dent Res 71 (11) : 1836-1841, 1992.

13. Mattison. GD, Von Fraunhofer. JA, Delivanis. PD & Anderson. AN : Microleakage of Retrograde amalgams, J Endod 11(8) : 340-345, 1985.

14. Moodnik. RM, Levey. MH, Besen. MA & Borden. BG : Retro grade amalgam filling : A Scanning electron microscopic study, J Endod 1(1) : 28-31, 1975.

15. Narang. R & Wells. H : Experimental osteogenesis with decalcified allogenic bone matrix in palatal defects. Oral Surg Oral Med Oral Pathol J 37 : 153, 1974.

16. Omnell. KA : Electrolytic precipitation of zinc carbonate in the jaw - An unsual complication after root resorption, Oral Surg 12 : 846, 1959.

17. Owadally. ID, Chong. BS, Pitt Ford. TR & Watson.TR : The sealing ability of IRM with the addition of hydroxyapatite as a retrograde root filling, Endod Dent Traumatol 9 : 211-215, 1993.

18. Pissiotis. E, Sapounas. G & Spangberg. LSW : Silver glass ionomer cement as a retrograde filling materials - A study invitro, J Endod 17 (5) : 225-229, 1991.

19. Pitt Ford. TR, Andreasen. JO, Dorn, SO & Kariyawasam. SP : Effect of various zinc oxide materials as root-end filling on healing after replantation, Int Endod J 28 : 273-278, 1995.

20. Rud. J, Munksgaard. EC, Andersen.JO, Rud. V. & Asmussen.I : Retrograde root filling with composite and dentin - bonding agent. Endod Dent Traumatol 7 : 118-125, 1991.

21. Saunders. WP, Saunders.EM & Gutmann.JL : Ultrasonic Root-end preparation, part 2 Microleakage of EBA root-end fillings, Int Endod J 27 : 325-329, 1994.

22. Schawrtz. SA & Alexander. JB : A comparison of leakage between silver-glass ionomer cement and amalgam retrofillings. J Endod 14 (8) : 385-391, 1988.

23. Sikri. VK & Poonam.S. : Attainment of hermetic seal with decalcified allogenic bone matrix grafts - Surgical Vs Conservative approach. J FODI 1(2) : 6-10, 1990.

24. Stabholz. A, Shani.J, Friedman. S & Abed. J : Marginal adaptation of retrograde fillings and its correlation with sealability. I Endod 11: 218-223, 1985.

25. Stabholz.A : Effects of Nd:YAG laser on apical seal of teeth after apicoectomy and retrofill. J Endod 18 (8) : 371-375, 1992.

26. Subba Rao. CV & Ramachandran.G : Book on Materials used in Dentistry, Chapter -3, : Pg 11-19, 1996. Sponsored by TN Dr. MGR Medical University.

27. Subba Rao.CV, Vimala.N & Kavitha. M : Book on microflora of oral Cavity, Chapter 15 : Pg 211-218, 1997 sponsored by Sree Balaji Dental College & Hospital, Co-sponsored by TN Dr. MGR Medical University.

28. Sumi. Y, Hattori. H, Hayashi. K & Ueda. M : Titanium inlay. A new root-end filling material. J Endod 23 (2) : 121-123, 1997.

29. Torabinejad.M, Smith. PW, Kettering.JD & Pitt Ford. TR : Comparative investigation of marginal adaptation of mineral

trioxide aggregate and other commonly used root-end filling materials. J Endod 21 (6) : 295-299, 1995.

30. Torabinejad.M, Hong.CU, MCDonald.F & Pitt Ford. TR : Physical and chemical properties of a new root-end filling material. J Endod 21 (7) : 349-353, 1995.

31. Torabinejad.M & Pitt Ford. TR : Root-end filling materials - a review. Endod Dent Traumatol 12: 161-178, 1996.

32. Vignaroli.PA, Anderson. RW & Pashley.DH : Longitudinal evaluation of the microleakage of dentin bonding agents used to seal resected root apices, J Endod 21 910) : 509-512, 1995.

33. Waikakul. A & Punwutikorn.J : Gold Leaf as an alternative retrograde filling material, Oral surg Oral med Oral pathol J 67: 746-749, 1989.

34. Waikakul. A & Punwutikorn.J : Clinical study of rerograde filling with gold leaf : comparison with amalgam, oral surg oral med oral pathol J 71 : 228-231,1991.

35. Walls.AWG : The properties of glass polyalkeonate (lonomer) cement incorporation sintered metallic particles, J Dent Mat 3 : 113-116, 1987.

A COMPENDIUM ON TITANIUM - THE WONDER METAL

Sukumaran V.G.

TITANIUM - THE WONDER METAL

The alloys and metals commonly used for military/aerospace, naval applications during the world war II could not withstand the high temperatures of jet engines and stresses produced by airfriction at great speeds. This lead to aggressive search for one such metal that would meet the specific needs. It was not until 1950 a wonder metal called Titanium developed, through the novel method of reduction which made a significant break through when it was successfully used in gas turbine engines for industrial purpose. It was found to be a light weight, high strength and excellent corrosion resistant metal. This led to the development of high altitude missiles, air crafts that flew faster than the speed of sound, under water pipes & valves and naval applications. Hence the story of Titanium and its alloys is an intriguing one, replete with the boom and bust cyclic fluctuations associated with material science largely tied to aerospace, naval / military applications. Its bio-compatibility and bio-functionality has led to its use as human body implants since 1980.

HISTORY OF TITANIUM

Titanium was discovered by William Gregor of England in 1791 and was named by Martin H.Klaproth of Germany in 1795. Titanium and its value remained a mystery until after the World War II because pure metal was almost impossible to obtain. During the smelting of ores the hot, molten mass absorbed atmospheric gasses and yielded a fragile useless product.

The first good process for metalic titanium was developed by the United states Bureau of mines. It used the Kroll's process invented by a refugee from Luxembourg, William Kroll. After a pilot plant produced the metal in tons, the U.S Government offered financial aid to provide companies to build a supply. Production rose sharply from 3 tonnes in 1948 to an annual average of more than 20,000 tonnes of sponge metal in the early 1980's.

ORES AND COMPOUNDS OF TITANIUM

Titanium is the ninth most abundant element in the earth's crust. The chief ores combine the dioxide with other elements. Rutile (TiO_2) is a mass of red to brown crystals of the dioxide with some iron. Ilmenite is a complex oxide of Titanium and iron ($FeTiO_3$).

Ores may be converted with highly concentrated Titanium dioxide or alloys of steel and other metals. It is as strong as steel but 45% lighter. It is 60% heavier than aluminium but twice as strong. It has very low heat & electrical conductivity and responds weakly to magnets. Such alloys are used in the production of missiles, space craft and high altitude aircrafts.

TITANIUM SPONGE

In the world 80% of the Titanium sponge is produced by the Kroll's process and only 20% by the Hunter's process. Electrolytic reduction process (Dow-Howmet process is now being practiced as well.

In the Kroll's process a mixture of Titanium dioxide (TiO_2) and coke are treated with chlorine to form Titanium tetrachloride ($TiCl_4$). This is passed through molten Magnesium forming Magnesium Chloride and sponge mass of metal. Titanium sponge is converted to Titanium metal products by a sequence of consumable melting operations and appropriate casting or deformation process - Titanium alloys can be got / cast. Hunter's process uses Sodium instead of Magnesium for the same process.

India possess more than 25% of the World reserves of Titanium. World reserves, (Thousand short tonnes of Titànium content).

Country	Total Reserves	%age of World Total Reseves
India	63,000	27.7
Brazil	38,000	16.7
South Africa	27,000	11.9
Australia	21,000	9.2
Norway	21,000	9.2
China	20,000	8.9
Canada	18,000	7.9
USA	8,100	3.5
USSR	5,600	2.6
Others	5,400	2.4
	2,27,100	

Defence Metallurgical Research Laboratory, Hyderabad (DMRL).

Demand Forecast for Titanium (EIL Survey)

End Use	Expected consumption in tonnes (1989-1990)
Aeronautical	80
Space Research	15
Chemical Industry	200
Power Generation	200
Petroleum and Petro Chemical	50
Electroplating	100
Heat Exchangers	50
Misellaneous	20
	715

World wide demand is currently oscillating between 25,000 and 35,000 tonnes per year.

IMPORTANT METAL CHARACTERISTICS

Titanium has a density of 4.50 Mg/m (0.16 lb / in) and titanium alloys have densities in the range of 4.50 - 4.84 Mg/m (0.163 - 0.175 lb / in). The density is considerably influenced by the alloy additions. High aluminium reduces alloy density. Pure titanium has ability to passivate in solutions and thus has exceptional aqueous (wet) corrosion resistance. This characteristic property is conferred on its alloys, though the alloys will not be as resistant as pure titanium. Titanium is resistant to oxidation upto about 593°C (1100°F) but it is a reactive metal that can pick up and dissolve interstitial elements like oxygen, nitrogen and hydrogen. Titanium has a very high melting temperature (1668°C 3035°F) but the allotropic transformation from the hexagonal close-packed (HCP) lower temperature to the body-centered cubic (BCC) high temperature form limits its application. Generally titanium and its alloys find use upto about 540°C (1000°F).

Titanium has an intermediate modulus of elasticity, 103 GPa (15.0 x 10 Psi). The modulus varies upto about 120 GPa (17.4 x 10 Psi) with alloys and can be varied by controlling the texture of the product. It has good ductility and can be not formed in a variety of shapes. Cold formability is restricted owing to the high spring back of titanium and a requirement for hot sizing.

Commercially pure titanium or unalloyed form is used in applications where optimum corrosion resistance is desired and where high strength is not a important factor. Oxygen functions as a controlled strengthener in unalloyed titanium. Strength increases as oxygen increases with in an acceptable range. Too much oxygen embrittles the material. Pure titanium is a base metal element but not a base metal alloy. There are six grades of commercially pure titanium but, generally only three are specified. The generally specified grade contain 99.01 tp 99.5% titanium plus small amounts of iron, carbon, hydrogen, nitrogen and oxygen. They are present in the form of residues which have significant effect on mechanical properties. Thus in the strict sense CP titanium is actually an alloy of titanium plus interstitial element. One grade also contain 0.15 to 0.20% Palladium for improved resistance to mildly reducing environment such as dilute hydrochloric acid and sulfuric acids.

Titanium alloys can be divided into three classes : alpha, alpha-beta and beta alloys. Additional phases are possible whenever heat treatment is done. The beta phase can transform to Martensite alpha phases on cooling. In addition, secondary phases can precipitate or be formed by deliberate alloy additions. Phases such as omega, alpha two (Ti_3Al) interface and gamma (TiAl) play a role in the properties of titanium alloys. Alpha two and gamma form the basis for potential new alloy systems.

The number of Titanium alloys commercially available are limited. The principal aerospace alloys are Ti-6Al-4V, Ti-5A1-2.5Sn, Ti-6Al-6V-2Sn, Ti-8Al-1Mo-1V, Ti-6Al-2Sn-4Zr-2Mo and Ti-13V-11Cr-3Al (Beta alloy).

Alpha alloys such as Ti-5Al-2.5Sn are slightly less corrosion resistant but higher in strength than unalloyed titanium. Alpha alloys retain ductility and toughness even at cryogenic temperatures, but cannot be strengthened by heat treatment.

Alpha Beta alloys contain one or more alpha stabilizers plus one or more beta stabilizers. These alloys can be strengthened by heat treatment or thermal mechanical processing. Generally when strengthening is desired, the alloys are rapidly cooled from a temperature high in the alpha-beta range or even above the beta transus. This solution treatment is followed by an intermediate temperature treatment (aging) to produce an appropriate mixture of alpha and transformed beta products.

Beta alloys are rich in beta stabilizers (lean in alpha stabilizers) that the beta phase can be completely retained with appropriate cooling rates. Beta alloys are unstable and precipitation of alpha phase in the meta stable beta is a method used to strenthen the alloy. Because of their high alloy content beta alloys are higher in density than alpha-beta alloys but strength density values of beta alloys may not be as high as those of the alpha-beta alloys.

Titanium undergoes an allotropic transformation from HCP (alpha phase) to BCC (beta phase) at about 882°C (1620°F). The transformation temperature is a function of alloy content and is strongly influenced by the interstitial elements like oxygen and nitrogen (as well as carbon). Some elements promote higher transformation temperature (alpha stabilizers) and others promote lower temperatures (beta stabilizers).

Physical properties of titanium show several interesting differences from the commonly employed structural metals. It undergoes a crystal transformation at 882°C. Above this temperature it has a B.C.C structure designated as Beta phase, while below it has a C.P. hex structure known as the alpha phase. This alpha phase has a c : a ratio of 1.587 - significantly lower than that for other hexagonal metals such as Magnesium and Cadmium. Thus there are more slip planes available fcr deformation. High purity Titanium is therefore a relatively ductile metal at room temperature. It can be deformed 95% or more between anneals. The phase transformation can be used to obtain a moderate increase in strength but at the expense of ductility. The commercially pure metal is soft enough to be readily cold formed and the higher strength alloys are easily forged. Machining is carried out with conventional machine tools but at a slower speed than is usual for most metals and alloys. Titanium and most of its alloys can be welded by argon-ARC technique.

Physical properties of commercially pure Titanium

Atomic number	Atomic weight	Crystal Structure		Melting point (°C)	Density (g/cm3)
		Below 882°C	Above 8823°C		
22	47.9	a = 2.9504A b = 4.683 A c/a = 1.587	a = 3.3065A	1660 ±10	4.51

Thermal conductivity ($W/m^{-1}k^{-1}$) at 20°C	Electrical resistivity (/cm) at 20°C	Specific heat ($Jkg^{-1} K^{-1}$) 0-100°C	Thermal expansion (20-100°C) (K)	Magnetic susceptibility 10-6cgs units^{-1})	Electrode potential w.r.t.sat Calomel (V)
17	48.2	528	7.6×10^{-1}	+3.43	-1.75

Mechanical Properties

The mechanical properties of titanium are affected by small amounts of oxygen and nitrogen in solid solution. It is therefore possible to produce a number of grades of commercially pure titanium with mechanical properties suited to the different applications for which the material is intended.

Mechanical properties of commercially pure Titanium

0.2% Proof stress (MPa)	Tensile strength (MPa)	Elongation on 50mm (%)	Fatique limit (% of T.S.)	Bend radius	Young's modulus (Gpa)	Density (g/cm^3)
130 - 460	270 - 740	30 - 15	50	1t - 21/2t	105 - 125	4.51

Compression

Titanium and its alloys are as strong in compression as they are in tension. Commercially pure titanium's compressive yield strength is about equal to tensile yield strength while Ti-6Al-4V and Ti-5Al-2.5Sn exhibit slightly higher strength in compression than in tension. Shear strength is 60 to 70% of ultimate tensile strength.

Hardness, rigidity and toughness

The hardness of commercially pure titanium is usually less than 120 Bhn for the highest purity grade. The hardness for other grades range from 200 to 295 for wrought material and 200 to 250 Bhn for castings. Ti-5A1-2.5Sn and Ti-6A1-4V have a hardness of 320 Bhn (340Vhn) in the cast condition.

Corrosion Behaviour

Titanium is intrinsically very reactive, reacts within microseconds to form an oxide layer whenever the metal is exposed to air, or to any environment containing available oxygen. A thin tenacious surface film of oxide is formed. This oxide, which is present on fabricated titanium surfaces at normal or slightly elevated temperatures has been identified as Rutile, a tetragonal form of titanium dioxide, and it is the presence of this surface film which confers upon Titanium a excellent corrosion resistance in a wide range of corrosive media.

The fundamental mechanism involved in the binding of the surface film to the substrate is not known with any certainty. According to the pilling - Bedowrth principle, the oxide formed at the surface of Titanium should occupy a larger volume than the metal from which it was formed, hence it will be compressively stressed. It is argued that thin compact films resulting from inward movement of oxygen, such as those formed on Titanium, are more protective than surface films formed by outward movement of cations. It has been pointed out that outward movement of cations may well leave vacancies at the metal oxide interface leading to a weakening of the bond between oxide and metal.

Nakayama, however has suggested that for Rutile, which is tetragonal in structure, the strong bond between metal and oxide results from the favourable spacing between Titanium ions in the Rutile lattice and those in the metal structure. This explanation however, does not account for the fact that other oxides of Titanium such as brookite, which is orthorhombic and, anatase, which is tetragonal are also protective. Another significant observation is that protective films on Titanium appears usually to be formed when the metal surface has access to water, even though this may be present only in trace quantity and in vapour firm. Its resistance to corrosion in sea water is relatively unsurpassed.

Chemical Environment

There is ample eivdence to suggest that in aqueous liquid environment the presence of an oxidising species, possibly coupled with the presence of hydroxyl ions, result in the formation of passive films at the surface of Titanium. Thus Titanium is very resistant to corrosion in nitric acid at room temperature, and at boiling point. Titanium has a significant corrosion rates in acids that normally produce hydrogen on reaction with metals e.g. Sulphuric acid, and Hydrochloric acid. The addition of small amounts of oxidising reagent results in the formation of passive films. Hydrofluoric acid, and Oxalic acid causes corrosion of Titanium becuase they form soluble complex salts with Titanium. Dry chlorine attacks Titanium but is resistant to wet chlorine. It has excellent resistance to all concentration of Nitric acid, Chromic acid and sea-water. At temperatures above 200°F (366 °K) Titanium may experience crevice corrosioin in Sea water and bromine.

Titanium is almost invariably resistant towards neutral salts, particularly halides at temperatures upto 100°C, and in respect to the latter environments it is significantly more resistant than stainless steel. In strong solutions of caustic alkalis, on the other hand, Titanium tends to form soluble Titanates, and is not resistant as nickel. In moderate or low concentration of alkali there is no significant attack, and the metal has appreciable solubility in concentrated or molten caustic alkali. It is resistant to attack by aqueous ammonia at all concentrations, temperatures and to anhydrous ammonia. Excellent resistance to corrosion in most organic acids with exception to Formic acid of about 10% concentration. In Citric acid of 50% strength at 100°C and Trichloro acetic acid there is significant corrosion. It is also resistant to mercury upto 150°C.

Resistance to Erosion

Titanium has outstanding resistance to erosion resulting from the presence of abrasive particles entrained in cooling water and process liquors. As a turbine blade material is subjected to impingement by water droplets moving at very high speeds, Titanium has been shown to be superior to other conventional steels virtually unmarked for 15 years.

Resistance to Crevice Corrosion

More resistant to crevice corrosion than most other metals and alloys particularly where differential aeration is involved e.g. it is very resistance to crevice attack in sea water at normal temperature. Crevice corrosion becomes more severe when acidity develops in the crevice and is more prone to occur under conditions of heat transfer. This can be avoided by coating with noble metals.

Titanium in Contact with other metals

In most environments the potentials of passive titanium, monel and stainless steel are similar, so galvanic effects do not occur when these metals are connected. Titanium usually functions as an efficient cathode and thus its contact will not lead to significant attack but can cause adverse galvanic effects upon other metals.

Resistance to stress Corrosion Cracking

CP Titanium is very resistant to stress-corrosion but fails when alloyed with aluminium. Specific environment to be avoided like pure methanol and red fuming nitric acids. 2% water in both these environments will inhibit cracking. On the contrary the presence of either bromine or iodine in methanol aggravates the effect.

Resistance to fatigue and Corrosion fatigue

The resistance of Titanium to fracture by fatigue induced by imposition of rapidly reversing stresses compares favourably with that of the more conventional metals and alloys. Commercially pure Titanium has a definite fatigue limit in air, about half its tensile strength, and at this figure, fracture may take place between 10^7 and 10^8 reversals. In this respect the commercially pure metal resembles steel. The fatigue limit for Titanium wetted with sea water is very similar to the figures obtained in air.

High Temperature Behaviour

Commercially pure Titanium is an established material for use at the moderately elevated temperatures attained in air craft exhaust shrouds and firewalls, but, neither titanium alloys are suitable at really high temperatures. The tensile strength of CIP Titanium shows a steady fall with increase in temperature. The tensile strength at 350°C being approximately half that at room temperature. The creep strength is improved by suitable alloying. An alloy containing 8% Al, 4.5% Sn, 4% Zr and smaller quantities of NB, MO, SI has a high creep strength at temperatures upto 600°C.

Above 600°C penetration of oxygen and nitrogen occurs. These elements make titanium brittle.

Casting

Titanium and its alloy castings are produced only by two processes, rammed graphite or investment casting. Alloys commonly cast include CP, Ti-6Al-4V, Ti-5Al-2.5SN and Ti-0.20Pd. Major uses are in processing industry and jet engines, air frame applications, medical and dental purposes. Rammed graphite mold castings upto 1500 lbs (680 Kg) and measuring approximately 36 x 72 in (9.4 x 18.28 mm) have been produced. Investment casting are generally used for small components.

Powders

Unalloyed and Titanium powders are now commercially available. They are produced by mechanical attrition, gas attrition, chemical attrition, hydride and communition from the molten states. Alloy powder can be produced by mixing elemental powders. The cost associated with powder metallurgy are very high.

USES OF TITANIUM AND TITANIUM ALLOYS

Used in air craft gas turbines, steam turbines, air craft skins, air craft body structures, an experimental submarine body, air craft landing gear, space craft structures, chemical or petrochemical heat exchangers, electrodes in fuel cells, anodes chlorine generation vessels to contain reactive chemicals, chemical pumps, helicopter rotor assemblies and medical and dental implants and prosthesis.

Medical and Dental Uses :

Joint Replacements

Cardio vascular systems - Mechanical heart valves
Cardiac Pacemakers

Artificial Pancreas - Open loop systems, Implantable pumps, constant rate pumps.

Oral and Maxillofacial surgery - Direct replacement of missing teeth e.g. Various types of Endosseous implants, implant in TMJ surgery, Reconstruction following tumour surgery, to assist in fracture Healing. Endodontics, Conservative Dentistry, Orthodontics, and Prosthetic dentisry.

MATERIAL DEGRADATION

The environment of the human body may be appear at first sight to be particularly aggressive. It is an aqueous environment, extremely well buffered so that the pH is maintained at around 7.4 at a constant temperature of 37°C. Degradation process can be considered to have both active and passive modes. The passive modes of degradation probably occur through mechanisms which are no different to those which occur in other non-physiological environments. The active modes are different, though it is difficult to say whether totally new mechanisms are operative or whether it is the kinetics of the various processes which are changed.

The role of active physiological environment in metalic corrosion is difficult to establish. It is known that the corrosion rate of some metals in saline can be radically altered by the presence of proteins (Clark and Williams, 1982). It is doubtful whether Titanium or Chromium based alloys, which are so strongly protected by an oxide layer, are significantly influenced by these proteins. On the other hand there are interesting theories and some evidence that some of the products of cell activation may be responsible for the development of the interfacial layer with Titanium implants. Tegvall et all (1989) for example have discussed the role of super oxide (O) generated by inflammatory cells in the production of hydrogen peroxide, in a reaction catalysed by the enzyme superoxide dismutase, on the oxide surface of Titanium.

SURFACE CHARACTERISATION

Implant materials should not adversely affect local tissues, organ systems, organ functions while in vivo environment should not degrade the implant and compromise its long term function. The interface zone between an implant and the surrounding tissues is therefore the most important entity in defining the biological response to the implant and the response of the implant to the body. (Albrektsson et al 1983)

The success of any implant is dependant on its bulk and surface properties at the site of implantation, tissue trauma during surgery and motion and the implant / tissue interface. The role of surface analysis in implantology is to : 1. Characterise the materials 2. Determine the structural and composition changes occuring during processing 3. Identify biologically induced surface reactions 4. Analyse the effects of the environment on the interfaces (Ducheyne and Healy 1988). It should be noted that the surface of a material is mostly always different in chemical composition and morphology than the bulk material. These differences arise from the molecular arrangement, surface reactions and contamination (Ratnar et al 1987). In this regard the interface chemistry is determined, primarily by the properties of the metal oxide and not as much by the metal itself. There is little or no similarity between the properties of the metal and properties of the oxide (Kasemo 1983), but the adsorption and desorption phenomena can still be influenced by the properties of the underlying metal (Healy & Ducheyne 1990). Therefore, characterisation of the surface composition, binding state and morphorogy are all important in the analysis of implant surface and implant/tissue interfaces.

Metallic oxide dictates the type of cellular and protein binding at the implant surface. Surface oxides are continuously altered by the diffusion of oxygen, hydroxide formation and the outdiffusion of metallic ions.

The surface potential may play an important role. It was postulated that oxides with high dielectric constants inhibit the movement of cells to the implant surface. Thus, the same authors suggest that one of the reasons for the positive biological response elicited by Titanium may be its high dielectric constant (Albrektsson et al 1983).

The mechanical state of the surface is also important. Macroscopic roughness, such as grit blasted, plasma sprayed or porous coated surface provides a better attachment strength between the implant and tissue or between the implant and PMMA or ceramic coating (Bobyn et al 1980).

Several recent studies have also addressed the concept of microroughness. Inone et al 1987 demonstrated that the type and orientation of cells attaching to the Titanium surfaces is influenced by the geometrical configuration of the substrate surface.

Chehrondi et al (1989, 1990) reported that epithelial down growth was accelerated on surfaces with vertical grooves and inhibited on surfaces with horizonatal grooves. Most important is the fact that these may not be singularly optimal surface for all types of cells and functions. It is unclear, however, whether the observations of cellular attachments on the surfaces of different roughness are truly a function of surface roughness or a function of alterations in surface chemistry encumbered during surface preparation.

METAL ION RELEASE FROM CP TITANIUM AND TITANIUM-6AL-4V IMPLANTS

The pioneers in the use of CP titanium implants, occasionally noticed blackening in the tissues surrounding the Implant. This indicates Titanium leakage from the Implant. No adverse tissue effects of the leakage have been demonstrated. Woodman et al inserted Titanium based fibre metal composite segmental bone replacements in the long bones of baboons. Metal concentration were measured in the lung, kidney, spleen, liver, muscle and in the lymph nodes adjacent to the implant in test animals for 8 years. In animals in which Ti-6Al-4V was inserted, Titanium levels were found to increase in the lung tissue of test animals upto 3 years. Thereafter a plateau phase was reached without further increase in Titanium levels. No evidence of any biochemical or hematological toxicity after 8 years, but they stated that the long term effect has to be observed. They also stated to study the neurological toxicity of aluminium and severe toxicity of vanadium. Owing to this reason, many a time commercially pure Titanium is used as human implant except in the joint/hip bone replacement.

CONCLUDING COMMENTS

This compendium has been attempted to highlight the salient and important characteristic of Titanium as a valuable metal. With advanced technology, biological understanding and sophisticated engineering it is apt to refer to Titanium as "the wonder metal" of the century, as its applications continue to expand into various fields, although aerospace usage remains the largest.

REFERENCES

1. In Vitro bio-compatability, mechanical properties, and corrosion resistance of Ti-Zr-Nb-Ta-Pd and Ti-Sn-Nb-Ta-Pb alloys. Astno Ito, Yoshimitsu Okazaki. Tetsuya Tateishi and Yoshimasa Ito. National Institute for Advanced Interdisciplinary Reserch and Mechanical Engineering Laboratory Ministry of International Trade and Industry, Ibaraki and Titanium Metals Technology Department Kobe steel, Ltd., Osaka, Japan.

2. Bone Tissue Response to Commercially Pure Titanium Implants Blasted with Fine and coarse Particles of Aluminium Oxide. Ann Wennerberg, Thomas Albrektson - Department of Bio-materials/Handicap Reserch, Institute for Srgical Sciences Goteberg University, Sweden S-41390 Goteberg.

3. Material Science and Technology. A comprehensive Treatment. R.S.Cahn, P.Haasen, E.J. Kramer Vol.14.

4. Tissue Integrated Prosthesis. Osseointegration in Clinical densitry. Branemark /Zabar / Albrektson. Quintessence Publishing Co. In 1985.

5. Does Titanium Surface Treatment Influence the Bone-Implant Interface? SEM and Histomorphometry in a 6-month sheep study. Gey Huri / Karl Donath, Maurice Lesourd, Daniel Chappard. Dr. Daniel Chappard Laboratori Faculty of Medicine 49045 Anger Cedex France.

6. Titanium Intermettalics - Present and Future. James C.Chesnutt, James A.Hall and Harry A. Lipsitt. G.E. aircraft Engines, Cinicinnatti, Ohio 45215 - 6301. Allied Signal Engines,

Phoenix, Arizona 85072. Wright state University. Dayton Ohio 45435.

7 Cellular uptake of Titanium and Vanadium from addition of salts or furtting corrosion in Vitro. A.M.Maurer, K. Merritt and S.A. Brown. Department of Biomedical Engineering. Case Western Reserve University Cleveland - Ohio.

8. Mold filling of Titanium casting using investments with different gas permeability, Morten Syvernd. Hakon Hero NIOM, Scandinaviun Institute of Dental Materials, Haslum, Norway.

9. Experimental long-Term study of Titanium ions eluded from pure Titanium miniplates. Kazuhisa Bessho, Kazuma Fujimura and Tadahiko lizuka. Department of oral and Maxillo facial surgery, Faculty of Medicine, Kyoto University, Kyoto 606, japan.

10. Matthew J. Donachie Jr. Titanium and Titanium alloys. Source Book. American Society for Metals.

11. R. Trivedi, J.A. Sekhar, J. Mzumdar Proceedings of Indo-US Workshops organized by Defence Metallurgical Reserch Laboratory Hyderabad, India.

12. Philip's Science of Dental Materials Tenth Edition. Kenneth J. Anusavice.

13. Review materials for Endosseous Dental Implants. J.C.Wataha. Medical college of Georgia School of Dentistry, Augusta, Georgia, USA.

GLASS IONOMERS

THE MATERIAL OF THIS CENTURY

Suresh Chandra B.
Ninan Joshua
Lavanya Rai

EVOLUTION

Glass Ionomers represent a new landmark within dentistry. There is yet a material of the kind glass ionomer to be introduced into the list of dental materials available to the dental practitioner. The glass ionomer in some form or other has been utilized by dentists globally in every sphere of dentistry. The material is continuing to occupy the top priority status, the status which it enjoyed for almost the last two decades. The evolution of glass ionomers dates back to late 1960's, when restorative dentists were trying to replace silicate restorations. The first breakthrough came when Dr. Dennis Smith suggested the use of polyacrylic acid to replace phosphoric acid in dental cements. The early work on zinc polycarboxylate cement provided an excellent clinical background for what was to follow. John McLean working with zinc polycarboxylate cements stated that, *"first the material stuck to every thing and was even difficult to remove from one's finger."* The tenacity of the bond to one's skin even after washing made McLean realize that he had then on hand a truly adhesive water based material. Wilson and Kent unravelled the setting mechanism of these cements and opened up a new field of exploration and research. They established that the setting mechanism was an acid base reaction and that it was an ion exchange system in which metal ions were displaced from glass powder and reacted with the polyacrylic acid to form a polysalt. The laboratory of the government chemist then proceeded with a methodical investigation of improving the properties of the dental silicate cement. Alan.D.Wilson and colleagues in 1965-1966 examined cements prepared by mixing silicate glass powder with aqueous solutions of various organic acids including polyacrylic acid. The result was unworkable and sluggishly setting cement. The rest is history. One cannot compare by any values the cements of 1972 and cements of 1998. Wilson and Kent coined the term Glass Ionomer in 1972 even though the International Standards Organisation terminology is polyalkenoate cements.

McLean and Alan.D.Wilson in 1973 were responsible for inclusion of tartaric acid in liquid, and in came a chain of improved cements into the market. The first commercial product and clinically usable material was with the global dentists by 1976. First in 1976 and later in the nineties as well as in late nineties the material has undergone revolutionary changes.

The introduction of light cure glass ionomer cement by Antonucci and his co-workers in 1988 and its further development into a commercially viable cement by Mitra in 1989, was a progressive step in the direction of combining the advantage of composite and glass ionomer.

In the late eighties, Mitra introduced the visible light cured glass ionomers, and a chain of events that followed led to confusions in terminologies was, and still is an experience that is unforgettable. However, Mclean in 1995 settled the issue by redefining, reclassifying, renaming and regrouping the various glass ionomers in the global commercial market. But still the controversies are on. Richard J Simonsen wrote in 1995 in his quintessence editorial *" Don't confuse me, consistency please".* He urged the authors, reviewers, editors and manufacturers to minimize confusion in our dental market place by following the excellent suggestions of Mclean et al. The American Academy of Restorative Dentistry in their annual review on the selected literature attacked the nomenclature proposals of Mclean et al in 1995 on the grounds (a) that they are advanced by supporters of traditional glass ionomer compositions (which is both irrelevant and untrue) (b) that the new terms "Muddy the waters". Sidhu S.K. and Watson 1995 described Mclean et al's nomenclature as ".... timely and based on sound scientific knowledge" and the American

Journal of Quintessence International has adopted it for all its papers.

INTRODUCTION

Glass Ionomer cement or more rightly named as polyalkenoate cements, are a hybrid of dental silicate and zinc polycarboxylate cements. An unusual material with unusual properties. However an universal material. Four major advantages and several minor advantages branching from it. The material bonds chemically to dentin, cementum and enamel with high degree of reliability. A reliable material with reliable properties.

The material is highly biocompatible and friendly to pulp and associated tissues. Anticariogenic, since the material has inherent built-in slow fluoride release mechanism. The glass ionomers allow for totally sealed restorative margins in that they are chemically and micromechanically bonded to dental tissues as well as composite resins. Glass Ionomers are many times referred to as **man-made dentin** as well as **dentin substitute.**

The major clinical limitation with the glass ionomers are that they are often opaque and does not demonstrate an esthetic acceptability comparable to that of composite resin or ceramics. Wilson and Mclean described the setting reaction of these materials to be essentially an acid base reaction between the glass powder and poly alkenoic acid. Graham Mount stated that the major advantages arising from the combination of these materials and chemistry is the ion exchange between the cement and the tooth structure as well as the continuing release of fluoride ions during the entire life of the restorations. These properties are unique and distinguishably credited only to glass ionomers and is of prime value in controlling dental caries and maintenance of caries free atmosphere in the oral cavity. These cements are now unquestionably used in all spheres of dentistry, whether it be restoration, liner, luting, buildups, fissure sealing/filling, management of erosive lesions, rampant caries young/adult, root end restorations, access restorations, repair material, tunnel preparations, preventive restorations to name only a few situations. A dependable material with reliable properties. Peter Hunt 1994 declared at the second International Symposium on glass ionomer that the conference proceedings demonstrated that far from being extinct, glass ionomer technology is alive, vibrant and developing fast. He further categorically declared that the conventional materials give far better results than they are generally given credit for when used correctly and in the right situations. When used in non retentive cervical restorations, they seem to be the bench mark to test by. When used as a base they seem to be the safety net that save the early generation of composite restoration.

COMPOSITION AND COMMERCIAL DEVELOPMENT

The glasses used in glass ionomer powder are ion leachable glasses. The ionomer glasses are unusual, unlike most silicate glasses, they are decomposed by acids, an essential property for cement formation. Glasses contain aluminium. Aluminium can enter the silica network replacing silicon, thus confirming a negative charge on the network which becomes basic and susceptible to attack by hydrogen ion in the acid. Three essential constituents of glass are silica (SiO_2), alumina (Al_2O_3) and calcium fluoride (CaF_2). Glasses high in silica, more than 40% are clear and transparent. Increase in CaF_2 and AlF_2 increases opacity. The first formulation had silica 30% and calcium fluoride (CaF_2) 32.4%. This was the basis of chemical composition of original G-200 or ASPA-I.

Cement formation is also related to glass composition. Al_2O_3/SiO_2 ratio is crucial (1:2 or more by mass for cement formation). Only if there is sufficient replacement of silicon by aluminium to render the network susceptible to acid attack, will the cement form. The compressive strength also increases with increasing alumina content. But although it is achieved at the expense of translucency. The glass used by the manufacturers are generally more complex. The types of calcium fluor alumina silicate glasses that may be employed in glass ionomer cement formation are listed below in increasing order of complexities (1) SiO_2 - Al_2O_3

- CaF_2 (2) SiO_2 - Al_2O_3 - CaF_2 - $AlPO_4$ (3) SiO_2 - Al_2O_3 - CaF_2 - $AlPO_4$ - Na_3AlF_6.

Glasses are prepared by mixing together the finely ground constituents melted in a sillimanite crucible between 1,100°C to 1,300°C for 40 - 150 minutes in an electric furnace. The melt is shock cooled by pouring on a steel tray. When the mass appears dull red it is plunged into water. The glass frit so obtained is ball milled passing through a sieve mesh with openings of dimensions depending on the required particle size for luting or for restoration.

Probably the modern so called transparent glasses have the following compositions, SiO_2 - 41.9%, AlO_3 - 28.6%, AlF_3 - 1.6%, CaF_2 - 15.9%, NaF - 9.3%, $AlPO_3$ - 3.8%.

The liquid consists of a co-polymer of acrylic acid, itaconic acid or co-polymers of maliec or tri carboxylic acids. Some formulations may also contain co-polymers of butendoic acid. Tartaric acid, a chelating agent is added to all glass ionomer liquid formulations. With the addition of tartaric acid, Willson and Crsip (1973) could convert a sluggish setting to a sharp setting cement with workable characteristics. These newer materials could be finished within 3-6 minutes or 7-15 minutes of cement formation. Co-polymers of itaconic acid and polyacrylic acid were developed to improve the shelf life by preventing hydrogen bonding and premature cross linking of acids.

Several powder and liquid formulation ratios have been suggested, but this depends on the specific indications of the cement.

SETTING REACTION

The setting reaction of the conventional chemically curing cements is not very well understood. However, the literature review indicates that these cements set probably in five clear cut stages.

(1) Decomposition of the glass and release of cement forming ions ; Calcium and Aluminium

(2) Migration of these metal ions into the aqueous phase of the

cement.

(3) *Gelation of the polyacid by the metal ions leading to cement formation*

(4) *Post set hardening begins when the metal ions get increasingly bound to the polyacid chain*

(5) *Further slow maturation*

Composition of the set cement is a highly complex composite. Then a cored filler is bound together by a hydrogel, by calcium and aluminum polyacrylates that contain fluoride, probably the end product is a fluor aluminum polyacrylate.

The stages of setting reaction of glass ionomers have very clear cut clinical significance. When the powder is brought into contact with liquid, the released metal ions enter into the aqueous phase and a bright shiny surface appears. At this stage mainly the calcium ion bridging is begining to form and the material is soft with the bright shiny surface. The material has to be utilized either for luting or for restoration or for any other purpose before the cloudiness sets in. Once the cloudiness sets in that means that there are no more COOH groups are available for bonding to dentin. Material at this stage can be cut like butter with a sharp instrument. Further when the aluminium ion bridging is completed the material sets to rock hard consistency.

CLASSIFICATION

A. *The following classification is adapted from Wilson and Mclean (1988). It is generally accepted.*

Type 1: Luting Cements

For cementation of crowns, bridges, inlays and orthodontic appliances.

Powder/liquid ratio approximately 1.5:1.

Fast set with early resistance to water uptake

Ultimate film thickness 25 µm or less.

Radiopaque.

Type II: Restorative Cements

1) Restorative aesthetic - auto cure and dual cure

For any application requiring an aesthetic restoration; the only limitation is no undue occlusal load.

Powder/liquid ratio 2.8:1 to 6.8:1

Excellent shade range and translucency

Auto cure cements have a prolonged setting reaction and remain subject to water loss and water uptake for at least 24 hours after placement; they require immediate protection from the oral environment

Most auto cure cements are radiopaque.

2) **Restorative reinforced**

For use where aesthetic considerations are not important but a rapid set and good physical properties are required.

Powder/liquid ratio 3:1 to 4:1

Fast set with early resistance to water uptake; can be trimmed and polished immediately after initial set; remain susceptible to dehydration for 2 weeks after placement.

Radiopaque

Type III: Lining or base cements

Can be auto cure or dual cure

Can be used as either a lining or a base, depending on the powder/liquid ratio used.

Powder/liquid ratio 1.5:1 for use as a lining material under other restorative materials.

Powder/liquid ratio 3:1 or greater for use as a base or dentine substitute in combination with another restorative material.

Physical properties improve as the powder content increases

Radiopaque.

B. Types of Glass Ionomers: (According to usage)

Type I - Luting Agents

Type II - a) Aesthetic filling materials

- b) Bis - Reinforced filling materials

Type III - Liners, Bases and fissure sealants

(Includes the Light cure or dual cure cements)

Dual cure cements : (Mitra, 1989)

Principal resin component is HEMA (Hydroxy Ethyl Methacrylate)

P/L ratio 3:1

C. McLean et al 1994 - Classification

1. Glass ionomer cement

Consists of a basic glass and an acidic polymer. It sets by an acid base reaction between these components. The definition is preserved exclusively for a material consisting of an acid ,decomposable glass and water soluble acid that set by neutralization reaction. The virgin glass ionomer cement embraces two sub-groups:

1. Glass poly alkenoates
2. Glass poly phosphonates

2. Resin modified Glass Ionomers

Hybrid materials that retain a significant acid base reaction as part of their overall curing process.

A feature of these materials is that they will set in the dark, however the process is slower than conventional glass ionomers.

3. Polyacid Modified Composite Resins

Material that may contain either, or both of the essential components of a glass ionomer cement, but at levels insufficient to promote the acid - base cure reaction in the dark.

Advantages of Resin Modified Glass Ionomers:

1. Improved setting characteristics
2. Command cure facility
3. Rapid development of early strength.
4. Impervious varnish application not critical.
5. Repairs possible
6. Two to three fold improvement in adhesion

Disadvantages:

1. Setting shrinkage higher - 1 %

PHYSICAL PROPERTIES OF THE CEMENT

	Property	Range
1	Powder/Liquid ratio (g/ml)	1.75 - 3.0
2	Rheometric working time (in minutes) 23°C	2.0 - 5.75 min.
3	Setting time (minutes) 37°C	3.5 - 7.5 min.
4	Compressive strength 24 hrs (MPa)	125 - 200 Mpa
5	Diametral tensile strength 24 hrs (MPa)	8 - 13.5 MPa
6	Flexural strength (MPa)	10 - 40 MPa
7	Creep, 24 hrs (%)	0.25 - 1.3 %
8	Film thickness (mm)	18 - 25 mm

Properties of Filling Cements:

	Silicate Cement	Glass ionomer Type II	Metal Modified G I C	Resin Modified G I C
Compressive Strength				
(24 hrs)				
MPa	180	150	150	105
Psi	26,000	22,000	22,000	15,000
Dimetral tensile strength				
(24 hrs)				
MPa	3.5	6.6	6.7	20
Psi	500	960	970	2,900
Hardness (KHN)	70	48	39	40
Pulp Response	Severe	Mild	Mild	Mild
Anticariogenic	Yes	Yes	Yes	Yes
Solubility (ADA Test)	0.7	0.4	—	—

AN UNUSUAL MATERIAL WITH UNUSUAL PROPERTIES

Commenting on the new glass ionomer formulations, Hunt 1994 said despite their advantages in the last few years, traditional materials have come to be seen as somewhat outdated. The development of light cured glass ionomer has been appreciated so well. He stated that these new materials are inherently stronger and seen much more user friendly. Being less prone to moisture contamination and dessication. In short Hunt said that they are faster, simpler, safer and stronger. All overwhelming advantages to the practitioner. Peter Hunt warned that one must be careful, however, these materials are not all alike. On one end of the sprectrum they are little more than dilute, inferior composite resins with little or no fluoride release or inherent bonding potential. He concludes by stating that it seems essential not to stray too far from the original glass ionomer technology with a true acid-base 'cure in the dark' technology to give the fluoride release and adhesion. According to Graham Mount in his writings and in his keynote addresses, as well as in his continuing education programmes has pronounced, that the virgin glass ionomer are the only one's that set by acid base mechanism. Peter Hunt also cautioned with concern while discussing the new materials, Hunt stated that besides the inherent chemistry there are other concerns about the new materials. Just as for dentin-bonding composites, their resin chemistry depends to a larger extent upon the use of HEMA, which may be more sensitizing than is generally believed. There is also the inherent potential for hydrogel formation in the resin component, which may lead to swelling and long term softening of the material. Additionally they may not be as color stable as the traditional materials, because some of the old self-cure resin technology is back in the mix. Unlike the traditional glass ionomers, which have 100% conversion and which rapidly become inert, the light-cured materials are bound to have a small residue of unreacted resin components in the final set material.

A. Bio-Compatibility

The glass ionomer cements are bio-theraupetic agents. Their ability to bond chemically to tooth structure ensures that they provide an excellent marginal seal, thus eliminating secondary caries, while their slow release of fluoride acting as a reservoir confers resistance to caries. These materials are not only bio-therapeutic, but they are also bio active, because there is an active exchange of ions between the tooth structure and the restorative material.

The poly alkenoic acid and especially poly acrylic acid, even though it has a pH of 1.7 still is considered to be biocompatible to dentally related tissues. The possible reasons for the blandness of polyacrylic acid narrated by McLean and Wilson 1974, and further confirmed by Wilson and McLean in 1988 are:

1. Polyacrylic acid is a weak acid.
2. The molecules are large and, large enough that they cannot pass through dentinal tubules easily.
3. Even if these molecules pass through, the polyacrylic acid forms complexes with collagen in the dentin and prevents further passage of acid closer to pulp.

According to Wilson and co-workers (1985) fluoride is released from glass ionomer for a sustained period of time, at least for 18 months. But others believe that the fluoride may be released in the form of a slow release mechanism throughout the life of the restoration.

Lennort Forsten 1995, declared at the IInd International Symposium on glass ionomer, that the permanent anticariogenic, bacteriostatic and remineralizing effect of the fluoride release from conventional autocuring glass ionomer cement can be predicted. These effects have been confirmed by laboratory studies, clinical studies and experience in the field.

However, Ivar A Mjor 1996 in his preliminary report based on a survey, demonstrated that the clinical diagnosis of secondary caries was the most common reason for failure in glass ionomer restoration. This report received worldwide protest and immediate reaction from several scientists, clinicians and practitioners, Edward J. Swift from North Carolina questioned the appropriateness of the research design, amount of detail reported, the variability and reliability of the measures and the appropriateness of the analysis in his letter to the editor (QI). Edward further stated that the study of Dr Mjor provided clear evidence for their lack of efficacy as such it might be subjected to misinterpretation or over interpretation.

Graham Mount responded, if my "bright outlook for glass ionomer restorative material" is to be challenged, I would rather like the challenge to come from an article with greater depth and a better base for comment. The material presentation is entirely anecdotal and resulting conclusions must be regarded as of very little consequence.

Peter Hunt opinioned in 1994 that, recently there has been an unfortunate trend towards evaluating restorative results from a short term, esthetic view point. The modern glass-ionomer systems according to Peter Hunt not only fare well by these somewhat superficial criteria but also point the way to less destructive and more reliable ways of restoring carious teeth and seem destined to break the vicious cycle of repair and breakdown that has characterized traditional restorative dentistry.

Glass ionomer materials have potent fluoride release potential. The initial burst of fluoride comes directly after the acid-base reaction. Much of this fluoride passes directly into the adjacent tooth structure, causing a conversion of hydroxy-fluor-apatite. Following the initial burst, which is a long term steady release of fluoride that seems to prevent recurrent wall lesions developing around glass-ionomer restorations. In fact there is a "reservoir" effect. Glass ionomers are increasingly being appreciated for cervical restorations because they seem less plaque attractive than resin-composite systems. As we move from traditional glass ionomer to resin-modified material we may loose areas of these benefits.

B. Bonding to tooth structure

Glass ionomer is an universal material with universal properties. It is a dentin substitute and also termed as man-made dentin as mentioned earlier. Glass Ionomer bonds to any substance with which it can react. It bonds very efficiently to enamel and more so to dentin as well as cementum. It bonds very efficiently to base metal alloys but does not bond to pure metals like gold or platinum. Since it bonds to dentin very efficiently, it is a very useful day to day material for the practitioner. Dentin bonding of glass ionomer requires moist atmosphere. Moisture means the inherent dentin moisture and not the saliva contaminated dentin.

To achieve better bonding efficiency, one must dry dentin to receive glass ionomer but not dessicate the dentin. The surface of ionomers are likely to go in for dehydration if not protected by a lubricating agent or a protective agent. People have used from vaseline to enamel and dentin bonding agents as a protective for the post setting phase of the glass ionomer system. Presently it is indicated to use either the visible light cured enamel or dentin bonding system as protectives.

C. Bilayered Restoration

Glass ionomers are efficient base materials, under composite restorations. The conventional sandwich technique proposed by McLean with a basic concept of sandwiching the glass ionomer between composite restoration on one side and dentin on the other side has come a long way. More and more people are now utilizing fourth and fifth generation bonding systems that clinically bond composite resin material to the dentin. The present terminology however proposed, if and when glass ionomers are used as base material below composite resin, it is bilayered restoration. Since the terminology coined earlier is considered erroneous. In fact there is no actual sandwiching and simply there are two layers with glass ionomer on the inside and composite resin on the outside. Etching glass ionomer was proposed in the eighties hoping for a clean glass ionomer surface for mechanical bonding. However, later it was realized that nothing really happens by etching glass ionomer as far as bond strength is concerned. There is a possibility of a cohesive failure with in the structure of glass ionomer by etching. However this does not have any telling effect on the bond strength. Glass ionomers could be good dentin substitute under composite resin restorative with a clear advantage of restricting the quantity of composite material in a preparation and thereby reducing to a great extent the polymerization shrinkage of resins.

E. Wear Resistance

The material has poor wear resistance and the wear resistance values are comparable to that of silicate material. Hence the material is not to be used in stress bearing areas as a routine restorative material. A few general practitioners on the advice of manufacturers have started using or rather misusing the glass ionomers for routine Class I and Class II preparations

F. Aesthetics

Glass ionomer materials are second priority materials as esthetic anterior restorative materials. Glass ionomers when indicated in the anteriors is indicated with reservations. It is a suitable material for Class III hidden lesions, otherwise the glass ionomer restoration used in anterior teeth have to be followed up by composite veneering. There are clinical and invitro studies to indicate that the glass ionomers becomes stronger and improve surface texture as it ages in the mouth. However there are no clear cut evidence for improved esthetics or translucency of glass ionomers as they age in the mouth.

G. Glass Ceremets

Metal modified glass ionomers. Glass-metal powders sintered to high density which can be made to react with acids to form a cement. Simmons (1983) - Miracle Mix, McLean & Gasser (1985) - Glass Ceremets

- Attempted improvements of flexural strength

- Incorporation of silver-tin alloys, fibres or flakes [Bis-reinforced GI - Type II (B)]

- Ion-leachable calcium fluoralumino silicate glasses used in preparation of powder.

Ceremet cements differ from simple mixture of metal and glass powder. Metal powder is firmly bonded to glass powder by high temperature sintering.

High packing density - Low porosity - Burnishable - Improved abrasion resistance - Colour improved by addition of 5% Titanium dioxide

Liquid: 37 gms of copolymer of polyacrylic and maliec acids,

9 gms of tartaric acid, and

54 gms of later

CLINICAL PROCEDURES

Conditioning and dentin conditioners

Glass ionomers bond to unconditioned dentin or enamel but bonds better to conditioned dentin or clean enamel. In comparison, composite resins cannot be bonded to unetched or untreated enamel. Several conditioning agents have been proposed for conditioning dentin.

Surface Conditioning

Citric Acid 50%,

Simple cleansers,

Chelating polyfunctional carboxylic,

Phenolic acids.

Powis 1982: For improving adhesion to enamel and dentin suggested: 25% polyacrylic acid, 25% tannic acid and an active surface detergent Dodicin 0.9%.

Mount 1984 suggested - ideal requirements for surface conditioning:

1. Should be isotonic to minimise osmotic effects
2. pH 5.5 to 8.0 - be neutral
3. Non-toxic to dentin & pulp.
4. Compatible with chemistry of cement
5. Have water solubility and be easily removed.
6. Not deplete enamel and dentine chemistry
7. Enhance the surface chemically in preparation for bonding

Mineralizing Solutions

Isotonic solution - Application time - 2 minutes

Promotes mineralization of dentin and increases concentration of calcium & phosphate ions within the smear layer (contains $CaCl_2$ 0.2, KCl 0.2, $MgCl_26H_2O$ 0.5, NaCl 8.0, $NaHCO_3$ 1.0, NaH_2PO_4 H_2O 0.05 Glucose 1.0.

More effective with Zinc polycarboxylates

EDTA cleans surface by chelations

PRECAUTIONS AND CRITERIA FOR SUCCESS WITH POLYALKENOATE CEMENTS

1. The tooth structure to be bonded should be clear and dry, but no dessication.
2. Glass ionomers demands a good mixing and packing technique.
3. Glass ionomer must have a glossy appearance before application.
4. Glass ionomers need matrix and wedge application
5. Glass ionomers need immediate protection during setting in the post setting phase.
6. Fast setting ionomers after preliminary set can be cut with rotary instrument in a slightly moist field.
7. Moisture should be excluded during initial set of glass ionomer
8. When using polyacrylic acid as a cavity cleanser it should be labelled as *cavity cleanser*. (This means it is a weak 25% polyacryclic acid as compared to using polyacrylic acid cement liquid which can be in excess of 50%) and can be applied for 10 seconds, rinsed and dried.

INDICATIONS FOR USE

Restorative Material

Erosion/Abrasion lesions

Sealing/Filling occlusal pits/fissure

Restoration of decidous teeth

Class III lingual approach

Repair of defective margins in restorations

Minimal cavity, approximal lesions, buccal & occlusal approach.

Fast setting lining cement base

Lining wherever biologic cariostatic action required.

Dentin substitute

Sealing and filling of occlusal fissures.

Early signs of caries.

Luting cements

Fine grain versions

Useful in patients with rampant caries and as well multiple caries lesions.

Core build-up, sealing root surface for over dentures provisional rest.

THE EROSIVE LESION RESTORATIONS

Lesion presents usually with 2 types of finishing lines:

- 'V' shaped notch with knife edges
- Saucer shaped lesion with no clear margins

The class V erosion-abrasion lesion falls into two categories:

- Total restoration with glass ionomer
- Laminated glass ionomer composite restoration

The success of the class V glass ionomer restoration depends on 5 factors:

1) Geometry of the lesion: Minimum depth of 1 mm for bulk.
2) Thickness & structure of tooth: Well defined cavosurface margin . Mandibular incisors can flex more than maxillary incisors.
3) Cleanliness of dentin surface: Stress on clear surface

4) Wettability of G.I. cement: Avoid dry mixes.

5) Aesthetics.

Graham Mount 1994 recommends specific cutting instruments for preparations to receive Glass Ionomer.

Diamond Stones

a) Tapered stones for entering, defining: Intensiv 206

Small cylinder for entering: Horico FG 106 010

Very fine taper for fissures: Abrasive Technology MFS 201 MF 1

Steel burs, latch types

b) Tapered fissure bur TF XC 700: 38/010

Small round for caries removal: 1/011-1/016

Long-shank round: 1/012-016 ELA

Extra-long shank: Moller Pulp bur, Meisinger 191/120-180

CLINICAL PLACEMENT OF GLASS IONOMERS IN GENERAL

ISOLATION

Saliva Control

Moisture in the form of saliva

Sulcular fluid or gingival haemorrhage

Moisture impairs the visual assessment. may contaminate the pulp during caries removal.

Negatively affects physical properties of the material. Rubber dam, cotton rolls and restoration cords used.

Other Steps

Tooth preparation

Lining

Shade selection

Surface conditioning

Matrix

Insertion of cement

Initial set

Removal of matrix & protection of cement

Finishing

FINISHING AND POLISHING

Even though most Glass Ionomers available today are rapid setting variety, most clinicians advocate a time gap of 24 hours before the final finishing and polishing is done. However, initial contouring can be obtained with the help of finely granulated diamond instruments under water cooling. For the final polishing flexible pop-on disks with different gradations can be utilized. A word of caution while finishing glass ionomer restoration is that the entire procedure has to be carried out under moist condition. Since dry cutting can dehydrate the glass ionomer material and the entire restoration may collapse in course of time. At the end of finishing procedures as mentioned earlier, glass ionomer requires protection during the post setting phase not only at the initial finishing and contouring but also at the end of final finishing and polishing procedures. The most accepted protective is either the VLC enamel bonding agent or dentin bonding systems.

POINTS TO REMEMBER ABOUT THE BENEFITS OF GLASS IONOMERS

1. *Glass ionomer cements are a cross between silicate cements & poly acrylic acid cements. They are an aluminosilicate glass (with fluoride) powder mixed with a polyacrylic acid. Each of the components give the glass ionomer, properties that are beneficial to the patient.*

2. *The fluoride in the powder leaches out of the set cement or restorative material (as a core) and provides a surrounding adjacent dentin and enamel resistance to reccurrent decay.*

3. *The polyacrylic acid is the basis for the chemical adhesion of the glass ionomer to the tooth structure. The chemical bond to the tooth structure has been well documented in the literature.*

4. *The recommended uses of glass ionomer cement to achieve optimal results includes: a base or liner under restorative materials, luting cement and as a core material for a cast restoration where adequate tooth structure is remaining to help support the casting.*

5. *Because of the adhesive nature of glass ionomers, they are an ideal material to be used as a thin liner under composite resins or dental amalgam or as a thermally insulating base under deep cavity preparations, because they do not need undercuts to retain them.*

6. *An added benefit of glass ionomer fast set liners are their use under composite resins.*

7. *The etching of glass ionomer liner/base is no more done.*

8. *The composite resin will now be able to bond mechanically to glass ionomer base.*

9. *When adequate tooth structure is remaining, glass ionomer can be used to restore areas of the tooth that will be a core for a cast restoration.*

10. *If a portion of an amalgam or composite dislodges during tooth preparations for a crown, the fast setting glass ionomer can be placed in that area and will adhere to the dentin, there is no need for undercuts. It can also be used to blockout undercuts in crown preparations prior to making an impression.*

11. *Glass ionomer cements are excellent as luting medium. They are adhesive to dentin and have physical properties that are equal to or surpassing zinc phosphate cements.*

12. *There have been reports of post operative sensitivity following cementation with glass ionomer cements and before their use. A determination of the status of the tooth should be made. One should always protect areas that are close to the pulp with calcium hydroxide.*

13. *After the casting has been cemented the margins will have the protection of the fluoride from the glass ionomer.*

14. *Glass ionomer cement are useful as repair material.*

15. *However, the material worth looking into is a buffered system which should be added to the restorative armamentarium. This will solve the problems where solutions did not exist before.*

16. *Keep in view the advantages / disadvantages of conventional acid base setting glass ionomer, resin reinforced glass ionomers and polyacid modified composite resin.*

FUTURE OF GLASS IONOMER

John W. Nicholson et al 1997 in their review on glass ionomer in restorative dentistry clearly indicated that the new resin-modified materials will have a major role to play in the clinical use of glass ionomer material. If a resin-modified glass ionomer cement has adequate wear resistance and fracture strengths to survive in a primary molar for 6 - 8 years, these cements will replace silver amalgam for the treatment of such teeth. A high sounding prediction? Resin-modified glass ionomer luting cements probably will be the material of choice in future. Presently and in future for cementation of stainless steel crowns, space maintainers and individual orthodontic bands. This statement could also be true for cementation of precision cast crowns and fixed prosthesis to prepared permanent teeth. With the tremendous development in the area of resin-modified glass ionomer cement, one must not conclude that the original self hardening acid-base setting virgin glass ionomer cement will be obsolete.

CONCLUSIONS

John McLean concluded in 1994 that the interest by the manufacturers in resin modified glass ionomer cements is growing and the future for this material is bright, since there are so many combinations of glasses and polymers to explore. He further stated that one should not forget the possibility of making an inlay material ,since laboratory conditions free us from the discipline of mouth-curing conditions. Higher curing temperatures and pressure curing can be used to eliminate porosity and allow the use of higher molecular-weight polymers. McLean believed that if dentists are to replace amalgam alloys, it may be necessary to return to metal reinforcement despite the obvious objection to the metal colour.

REFERENCES

1. Alan D. Wilson, John N. McLean : Glass Ionomer Cements, Quintessence book, 1988
2. Buratieri, Luiz N. et al : Advanced Operative Dentistry, Glass Ionomer Cement Restoration, Quintessence book, 1993, 167-186.
3. Carel L. Davidson : Glass Ionomer Bases under Posterior Composites, IInd International Conference on Glass Ionomer, 1994, Vol.6, No.5, Journal of Esthetic Dentistry, 223-226.
4. Edward J. Swift, James D. Bader, : Glass Ionomer Cement Restorations and Secondary Caries (Letter Quintessence International) 1996, 27, 581.
5. Graham J. Mount, Daniel A. Shugars : Another letter on Glass Ionomer Cement Restorations (Letter Quintessence International) 1996, 27, 582-583.
6. Graham J. Mount : An Atlas of Glass Ionomer Cements - A Clinicians Guide, IInd edition 1994.
7. Ivar A. Mjor : Glass Ionomer Cement Restorations and Secondary Caries (A preliminary report,

Quintessence International) 1996, 27, 3, 171-174.

8. John Burgess, Barry Norling, James Summitt : Resin Ionomer Restorative Materials-The New Generation, IInd International Conference on Glass Ionomer, 1994, Vol.6, No.5, Journal of Esthetic Dentistry, 207-215.

9. John W. McLean : Evolution of Glass Ionomer Cements: A personal view, IInd International Conference on Glass Ionomer, 1994, Vol.6, No.5, Journal of Esthetic Dentistry, 195-206.

10. John W. Nicholson, Theodore P. Croll : Glass Ionomer Cement in Restorative Dentistry, Quintess -ence Inter-national, 1997, 28, 705-714.

11. Lennart Forsten : Fluoride release of Glass Ionomers, IInd International Conference on Glass Ionomer, 1994, Vol.6, No.5, Journal of Esthetic Dentistry, 216-222.

12. Loyd C.H. et al : Dental Materials Literature, Review, Journal of Dentistry, 1995, Vol. 25, 3, 4, 173-208.

13. McLean J.W., Nicholson J.W. : Suggested nomenclature for glass ionomer cements and related materials. Editorial Quintessence International, 1994, 25, 587-589.

14. Peter Hunt, Wilson A.D. : Glass Ionomers: The Next Generation, A Summary of the Current Situation, IInd

International Conference on Glass Ionomer, 1994, Vol.6, No.5, Journal of Esthetic Dentistry, 192-194.

15. Robert L. Erickson, Eileen A. Glass Poole : Bonding Tooth Structure: A comparison of Glass Ionomer and Composite Resin Systems, IInd International Conference on Glass Ionomer, 1994, Vol.6, No.5, Journal of Esthetic Dentistry, 227-244.

16. Richard J. Simonsen : "Don't Confuse Me Consistency Please" Quintessence International, Editorial, 1995, 26, 12, 827.

A CENTURY WITH CERAMICS

Susila V.

INTRODUCTION :

The word ceramics is derived from the greek word 'keramos' which means 'pottery' or 'burnt stuff'. Ceramics are the earliest group of inorganic materials to be structurally modified by man and his early history is principally traced through these materials. They are the first materials to be the subject of early laboratory research. The development of dental ceramics parallels the industrial revolution.

Early fabrication of ceramic articles dates back to 23,000 BC. Three basic types of ceramic materials were developed, 1. Earthenware 2. Stoneware 3. Porcelain. Porcelain is obtained by fluxing white china clay with chine stone to produce white translucent stoneware. Porcelain in english & many other foreign languages means 'china'.

HISTORICAL BACKGROUND :

Fauchard described the use of baked enamel as early as 1728 for esthetic purpose. In 1760, Fauchard, Bordet and other dentists constructed gum colour enamel and gum section teeth. In 1774, Alexis Duchateau constructed the first set of mineral dentures with the porcelain manufacturers of Guerhard factory, but firing shrinkage was more. Nicholas Duboius de Clement improved Duchateau's fabrication method. His original porcelain paste was made from 30 pounds of white fountainbleau sand 10 pounds of Alicant barilla. 7 pounds of this mixture was ground with 2 pounds of white marble and ground to produce a smooth paste. In 1838, Elias Wildman formulated translucent porcelain. In 1850, Samuel Stockton, S.S. White & Claudius Ash placed the porcelain tooth on a successful commercial basis. Dr. Charles H. Land filed the first patent for the porcelain jacket crown fabrication in 1889. The traditional porcelain was obtained from a remarkably pure marble mined at an island in the Algean Sea named Paros. This was extremely translucent. The parian China had feldspar as its principal constituent and developed a self glaze on firing. These ceramic materials did not have strict chemical composition corresponding to traditional chemical formulae. Later in 1907 Stockton developed dental porcelain with a mineral composition of :

Feldspar	-	78%
Kaolin	-	15.3%
Potassium Silicate	-	4.7%
Dehydrated Borax	-	2%

CLASSIFICATIONS OF MATERIALS:

Broadly Ceramics can be classified as :

1) Feldspathic Porcelain 2) Crystalline Ceramics

Based on their use they can be classified as :

1) Core Ceramics 2) Veneer Porcelains

Based on their method of fabrication they may be classified as :

1) Conventional porcelains using condensation and sintering
2) Castable Ceramics
3) Pressable Ceramics
4) Machinable Ceramics
5) Infiltrated Ceramics

Feldspathic Porcelain :

This is mainly used as a veneer over stronger core materials. This is the ultimate in aesthetic restorations. Of all currently available aesthetic restorative materials, this is the closest in match to enamel's translucency and shade. Virtually any ceramic material in itself cannot aesthetically match the natural tooth as well and hence requires the layering of feldspathic porcelain to achieve that end.

Feldspathic porcelain is sub divided into :

(1) High expansion porcelains suitable for veneering metals and magnesia core ceramics.

(2) Low expansion porcelains suitable for veneering other ceramics.

Depending on their fusion temperature they may be further sub classified as :

(1) High fusing porcelains used for manufacturing denture teeth.

(2) Medium fusing porcelains for all-ceramic restorations.

(3) Low fusing porcelains for metal ceramic and all ceramic.

(4) Ultra-low fusing porcelains for metal ceramic and all ceramic restorations.

Composition :

Dental porcelains use the basic silicon - oxygen network as the glass - forming matrix, but additions of other oxides to the basic SiO_4 lattice, like those of potassium, sodium, calcium, aluminum and boron impart properties like low fusion temperature, high viscosity and resistance to devitrification (ability to maintain the glassy nature)

The glass matrix of porcelain is supplied by the feldspar which is its major constituent. It is a natural mineral and is a precursor for clay. Geographical variation in the type of feldspar makes two types, Albite (Soda feldspar) and Orthoclase or Microcline (potash feldspar) available.

Quartz and a small quantity of kaolin complete the rest of the composition.

Colouring pigments : Metallic oxides provide the colour that is heat resistant. Chromium, tin or chrome-alumina provide pink hue.

This eliminates the greenish hue due to glassy nature. Praesodymium, Indium provide a ivory hue. Vanadium - Zirconium, Tin - Chromium also provide ivory hue but are not stable. Cobalt provides blue hue. Gray hue is provided by Iron oxide and Platinum which also imparts translucency.

Opacifying agents : Metallic oxides of Cerium, Titanium, and Zirconium impart opacity. The particle size should match the wavelength of visible light, 0.4 - 0.8 μm. This produces a blue tinge in reflected light but turn yellowish red in transmitted light resembling natural tooth.

Stains or colour modifiers : Stains are surface colorants used to produce check lines, decalcification spots in the body porcelain. Colour modifiers are used to obtain gingival effects or highlight body colours. Stains are pure metal oxides or lower fusion point glasses so that they can be applied at temperature below those of enamel and dentin porcelains. Colour modifiers are used at the same temperature as dental porcelain.

Fluorescing agents : The use of conventional sodium duiranate for this purpose has been banned due to radiation hazards. Samarium in 5 ppm or spinel can be substituted, though they are not as effective as uranium salts.

Glazes and Add on porcelains : The Glazes consist of uncoloured glass powders. A glaze should normally mature at a temperature lower than that of the restoration and its thermal expansion coefficient should be fractionally lower than the ceramic body. Add on porcelains are similar to glaze but for the addition of opacifying agents and colouring pigments. These are used for simple corrections of tooth contour and contact points.

The pertinent physical and mechanical properties are given in Table No.1.

Fabrication :

It is composed of two steps (1) Condensation (2) Sintering or firing.

Condensation : The process of packing the particles together and of removing the excess liquid binder is known as condensation. The mix should be thick and creamy in consistency. The main driving force involued in condensing dental porcelain is surface tension. The withdrawal of water from the powder will always cause the powder particles to pack more closely. High room temperatures and dry atmospheres are to be avoided since porcelain can rapidly dry out.

In the wet-brush technique, the porcelain mix is carried in a sable brush or le cron carver or spatula taking care that it does not drip off at the end. The mix should not be over-stirred as this might incorporate large air bubbles. This technique is also known as 'Brush additive technique'. The brush is used to flow the wet porcelain and a gentle pushing or tapping motion will agitate the porcelain particles into position and the brush will keep this porcelain moist. Excess water is withdrawn with a paper tissue and surface tension will automatically cause the particles to settle closer together. Vibration of the porcelain should be kept to a minimum as this may cause the material to slump. Whipping with a large brush is also detrimental. Such brushes are used only to smooth off the surface.

Sintering : Porcelain undergoes densification during sintering. The initial rate of sintering is inversely proportional to the particle size and viscosity and directly proportional to the surface tension. If air firing is done, a very slow maturation period is the ideal for which to aim is to allow the escape of maximum amount of entrapped air. During this procedure the porcelain must not be raised to its final maturing temperature, but 30°C-50°C below it. A heat soak of half-an-hour can often be safely contemplated.

In vacuum firing, it is actually air under low pressure. The air in the interstitial spaces is removed before the sealing of the surface occurs. When vacuum is released, air at normal pressure causes a strong compression effect on the dense outer surface, which compresses the low pressure internal residual air bubbles. This results in relatively dense, pore-free porcelain.

Diffusible gases like helium, hydrogen or steam can be used in place of air. These gases will be sealed in the interstitial spaces and such spaces do not enlarge with temperature, but decrease and disappear due to diffusion or dissolution.

Stages of maturity :

Low bisque : The surface of the porcelain is very porous and will easily absorb water soluble die. Grains would have started lensing at the contact points. Shrinkage is minimal but the porcelain is very weak.

Medium bisque : The surface is still porous but the flow of the glass grains will have increased and entrapped air will become sphere shaped. A definite shrinkage would have taken place.

High bisque : The surface is completely sealed and presents a smooth texture. Porcelain is very strong but grinding is possible.

Glazing : Self glazing is the most preferred technique. It is simply a further stage of vitrification from the bisque finish. This is done by increasing the time of high bisque maturation. Too high a temperature, increases pyroplasticity and loss of surface detail.

CRYSTALLINE CERAMICS :

ALUMINA & ALUMINOUS PORCELAINS :

Alumina is the hardest and probably the strongest ceramic oxide known. Alpha alumina is commonly used for ceramic applications. It is used in the form of prefabricated profiles or reinforcement for the construction of crowns, bridges or individual pontics.

As early as 1965, Mc Lean and Hughes developed aluminous porcelains for improving the strength of the material. Alumina crystals dispersed in the glass matrix prevent crack propagation.

Aluminous porcelains are available under various commercial names as Vita Dur, Hi-Ceram etc.

Composition :

ALUMINOUS PORCELAINS

40-80% of the material contains alumina crystals and the rest is formed by feldspar, quartz and kaolin. The proportion of alumina will vary depending on the intended use.

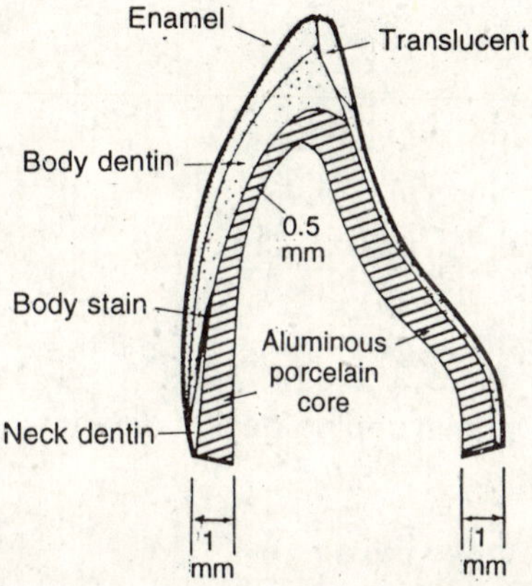

Fig (1) - Cross-sectional view of aluminous porcelain jacket crown.

Fabrication :

It is similar to feldspathic porcelain excepting that the sintering should be very slow to allow the porosity to escape at the grain boundaries. The porcelain should not reach the maturing temperature in less than 5 mts. It should enter the hot zone of the furnace at atleast 250°C below the final temperature. The rate of sintering should be 50°C/mt.

SHRINK-FREE CERAMICS :

These were introduced by Sozio and Riley in 1983. Conventional firing shrinkage is compensated by the reaction of the constituents crystals namely alumina and magnesia to form magnesium aluminate or spinel.

Composition :

It is an aluminous porcelain containing silicone resin which makes it mouldable at lower temperatures. This silicone converts into silica upon firing and combines with the alumina to form aluminosilicate. This in turn reacts with incorporated magnesia to form spinel, which is also one of the strongest ceramic oxides. Alkaline earth glass constituents like Ca and Be aid in sintering process and contributes to corrosion resistance due to the absence of alkali ions like Na, Li, & K.

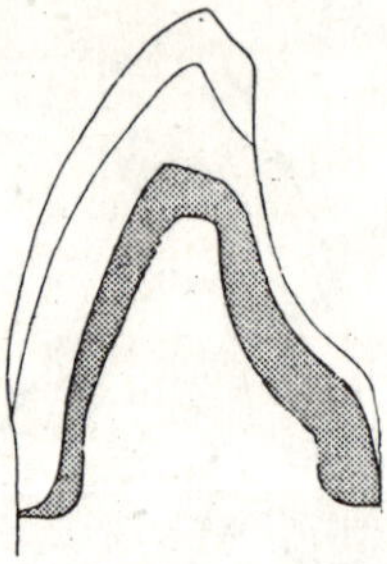

Fig (2) - Optimal coping design anterior

Fabrication :

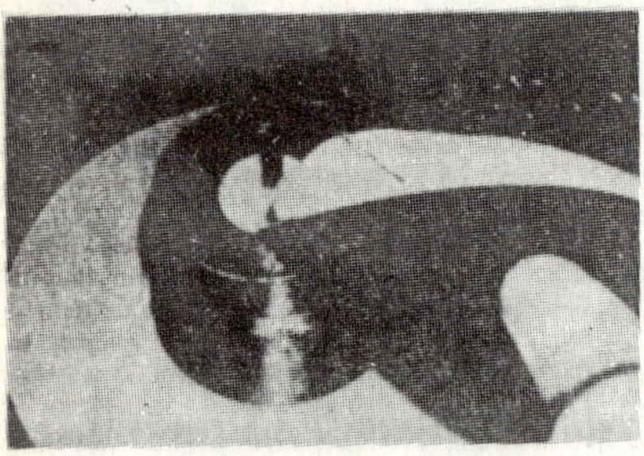

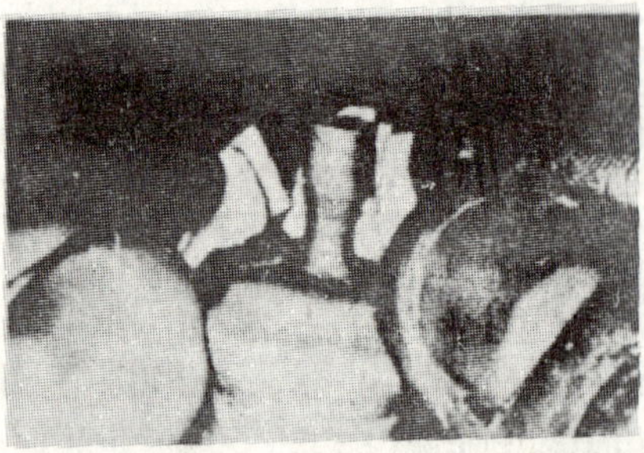

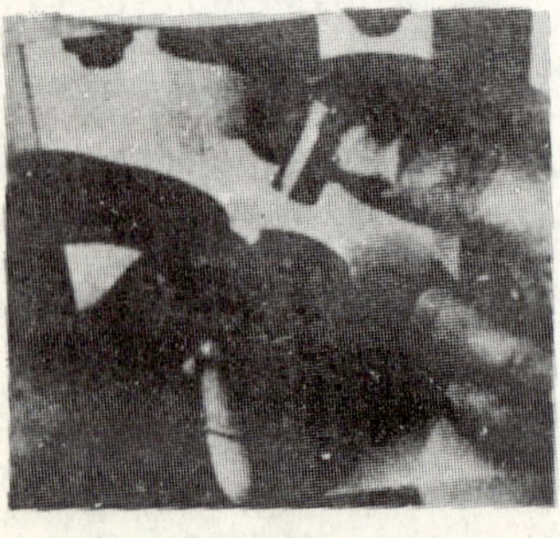

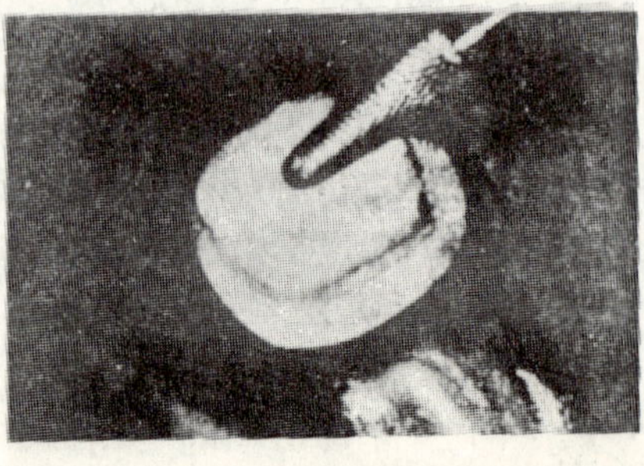

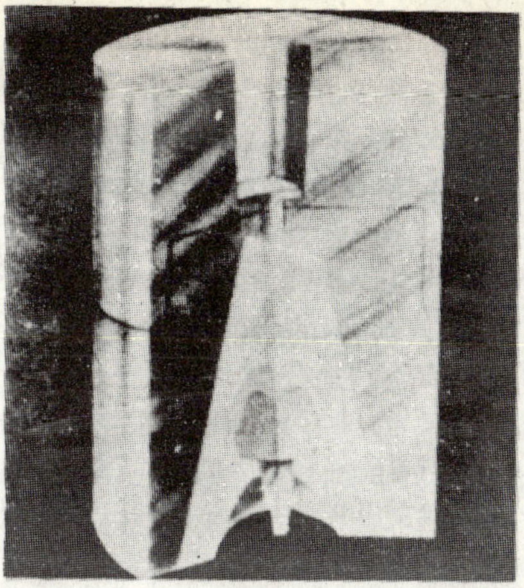

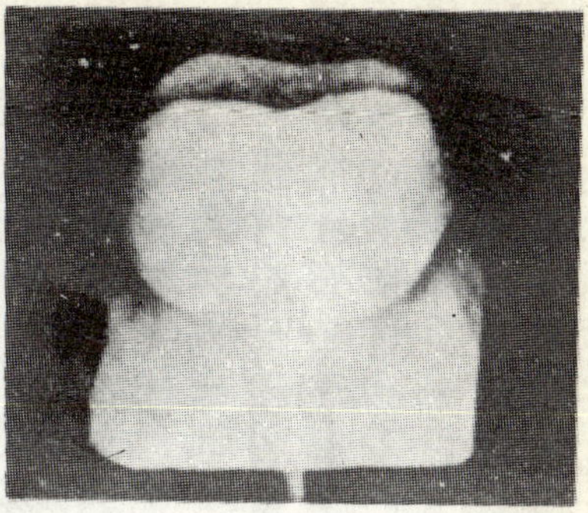

Fig (3-a) - Investing wax up on die with plaster Fig (3-b) - Plaster removal from pressed coping and master die. Fig (3-c) - Placing ceramic pellet in flask for pressing Fig (3-d) - Refining green state (unfired) coping Fig (3-e) - Cross-sectional diagram of ceramic injected into mold Fig (3-f) - Pressed coping (unfired) on master die.

Injection Moulding : A special epoxy die is prepared and wax up of the coping is done on it. It is invested in a flask with dental stone and plaster. The wax is boiled out and flask is heated to 180°C. The ceramic is transfer moulded into the cavity of the flask. The epoxy die is retrieved with the formed coping. The sprue is trimmed and the coping refined. It is then fired at 130°C in a controlled manner in a programmable furnace. Transition and veneer porcelains are added in the conventional manner.

Shrink - free ceramics were marketed as two generation of materials under the commercial names of Cerestore and Al-ceram respectively.

MAGNESIA CORE CERAMICS :

This is a high expansion ceramic. This can be used as a core for metal-ceramic veneer porcelains.

Magnesia is a face-centered cubic crystal and strengthens both by dispersion strengthening of the vitreous matrix and crystallization within the matrix.

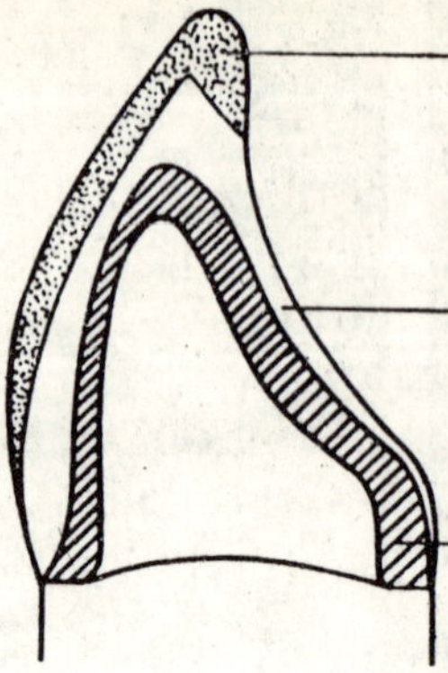

Fig (4) - All-ceramic crown made with porcelain fused to metal (PFM) type of translucent procelains over a high-expansion magnesia core material.

Fabrication is similar to conventional porcelains with the exception that this can be internally glazed. This internal glaze blocks the pores and doubles the strength.

GLASS CERAMICS :

These are castable ceramics introduced by Mc Culloch in 1968. These are based on the growth of in-situ crystals (both nucleation and crystallization) by a controlled heat treatment of a glass called 'ceramming'. Dicor, the commercial glass - ceramic was developed by Peter Adair and William Grossman in 1984.

Composition :

It contains SiO_2, K_2O, MgO, Al_2O_3, ZrO_2, a fluorescing agent and MgF_2 as nucleating agent in the glass. The micro-structure after ceramming consists of many small interlocking plate-like crystals of tetrasilicic fluoromica. This intersection of crystals causes crack deflection and blunting which accounts for its strength.

Commercially Dicor corresponds to this typical composition.

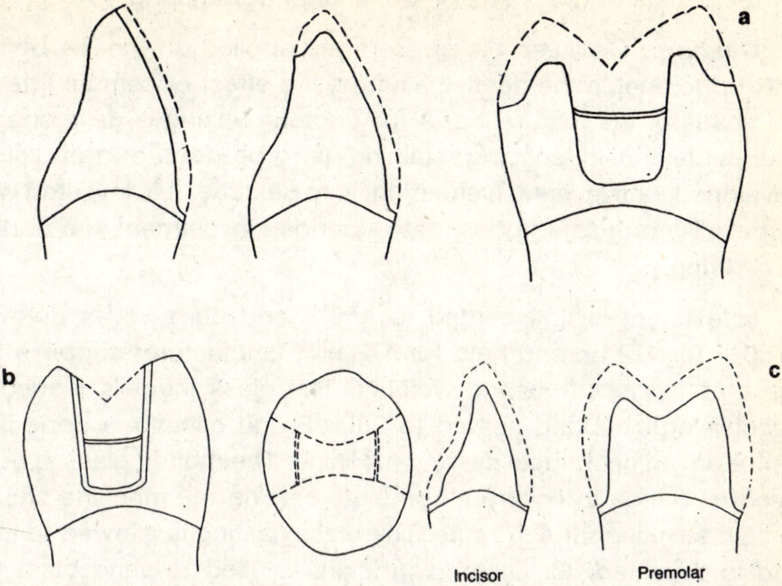

Fig (5) - Dicor laminate vaneer preparation form. Fig (5-a) - Dicor inlay preparation form. Fig (5-b) - Dicor onlay preparation form. Fig (5-c) - Full-veneer crom preparation form.

Fabrication :

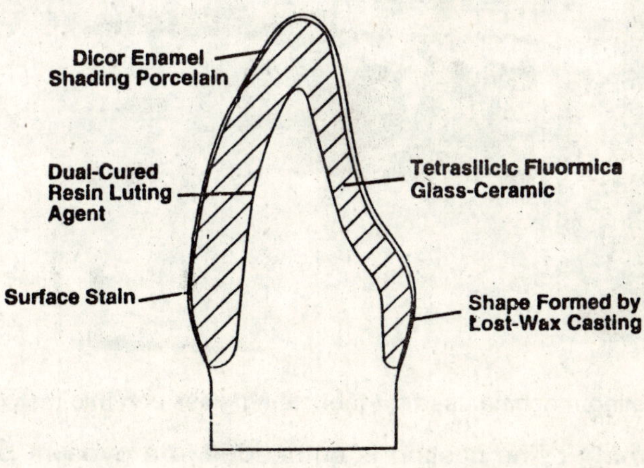

Fig (6) - Typical materials used in the construction of a Dicor glass-ceramic crown

It consists of two steps (1) Casting (2) Ceramming.

Casting : Coloured die spacers are applied on the die before wax-up to enable the dentist visualize the effect of cement lute on the shade of the restoration. A full contour waxing is developed if external (extrinsic) shading (staining) is to be done or a coping is developed, or if layering (veneering) is to be done. It is invested with a specially formulated phosphate - bonded investment in a double - lined ring.

Investment is first heated to 450°F and burn out is done at 1750°F for 1/2 hr. and held for 1/2 hr. Manufacturer supplies the glass as ingots of varying weights. The glass ingot is placed in Zirconia crucible and heated to 2600°F and casting is done in a motor driven centrifugal casting machine. The molten glass is quite viscous. Hence to ensure a complete casting the machine should remain spinning for 4 1/2 mts. The glass casting is allowed to cool and is devested. Al_2O_3 of 25 μm grit is used to sand blast the casting at 40 psi to remove the remnants of investment. The sprue is removed.

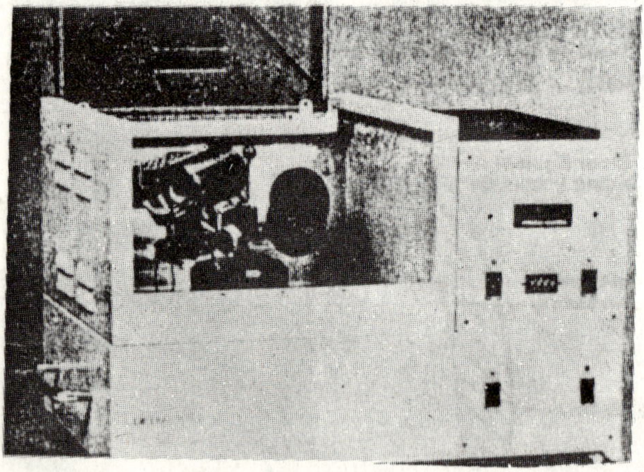

Fig (7) - Casting machine used for fabricating glass ceramic restorations.

Ceramming : The casting is embedded in a gypsum bonded investment and subjected to controlled crystallization. The cycle runs from 650°C - 1075°C for 1 1/2 hrs and sustained for 6 hrs.

Tetrasilicic floroamica ($K_2 Mg_5Si_8 O_2 OF_4$) forms as interlocked crystals in the glass matrix constituting about 55% of it.

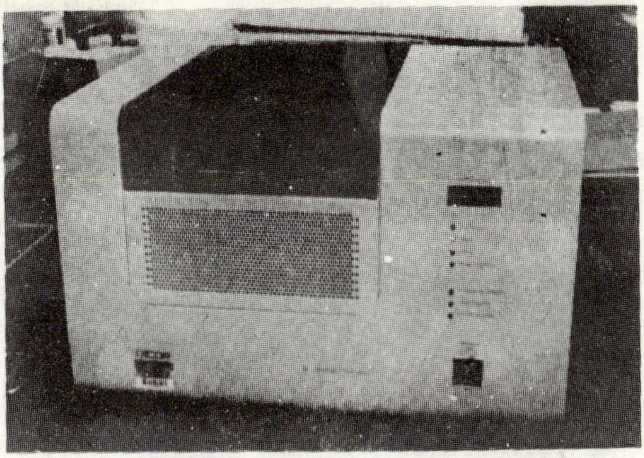

Fig (8) - Dicor® ceramming oven.

APATITE GLASS - CERAMIC :

Commercially available cera pearl is a development of a apatite glass - ceramic developed by Hobo & Iwata in 1985.

Composition :

It is a calcium phosphate which turns into oxyapatite on heat treatment. This upon exposure to water converts into hydroxyapatite.

Fabrication :

It is similar to glass-ceramics excepting that the ceramming is done at 870°c for 1 hr.

LITHIA BASED GLASS-CERAMIC

This was developed by Uryu. Commercially it is available as Olympus Castable Ceramic (OCC).

Composition :

It contains mica crystals of Na Mg_3 (Si_3 AlO_{10})F_2 and beta

Spodumene crystals of $Li_2 OAl_2O_3 4SiO_2$ after heat treatment.

MACHINABLE CERAMICS :

Industrial quality ceramic blocks are milled using CAD-CAM technique to give restorations that are pore-free and stronger. Though as early as in 1971, It was introduced, it was not until 1988 that it became popular. The first CAD-CAM unit marketed by Siemens by name Cerec meaning ceramic reconstruction, recommends 3 materials to be used for machined restorations.

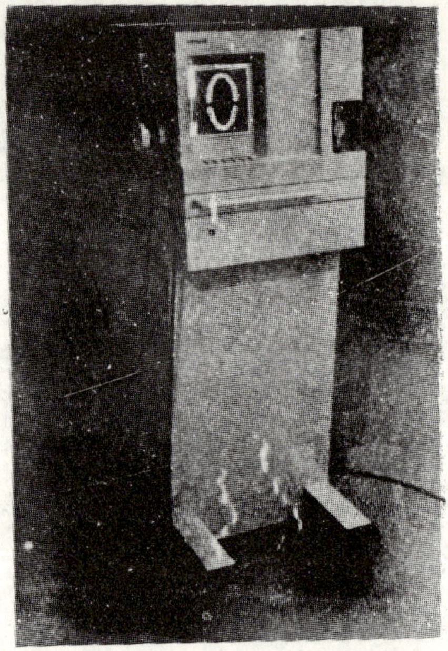

Fig (9) - CEREC® CAD/CAM device.

Cerec Vita blocs Mark I: This is the first material to be used in CAD CAM and is a feldspathic porcelain.

Cerec Vita blocs Mark II: It is a fine grained strengthened feldspathic porcelain.

Dicor MGC : It has higher strength values than Dicor.

CAD CAM Technique :

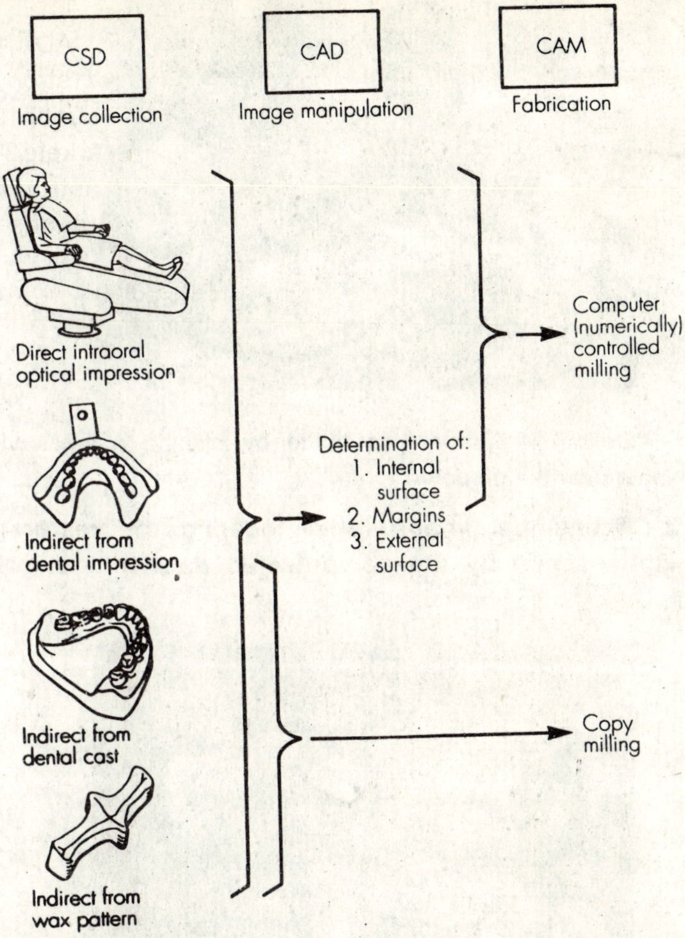

Fig (10) - Schematic summary of CAD/Cam and copy milling operations.

This uses digital information about the cavity preparation or a pattern of the restoration, to provide a computer - aided design. An intra oral infra red camera captures the image of the prepared and adjacent teeth which is displayed on the monitor of video for inspection and modification.

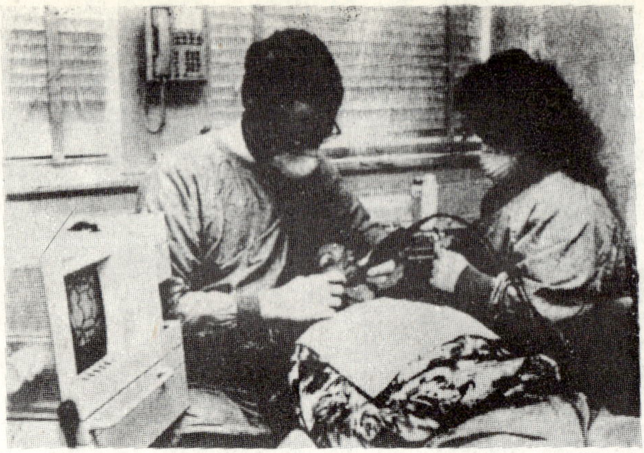

Fig (11) - "Optical impression" is made by placing a small video camera/scanner over the prepared tooth.

This 3-Dimensional image, after locating the restoration margins, is translated by the computer as data to the milling (CAM)unit.

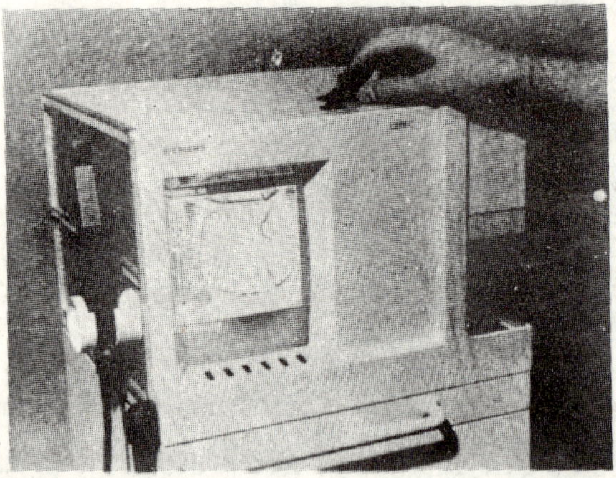

Fig (12) - Restoration is designed on computer screen by drawing position of gingival margins and proximal contacts. The device automatically finds the position of occlusal margins. Design time for experienced operator is 3 to 5 minutes.

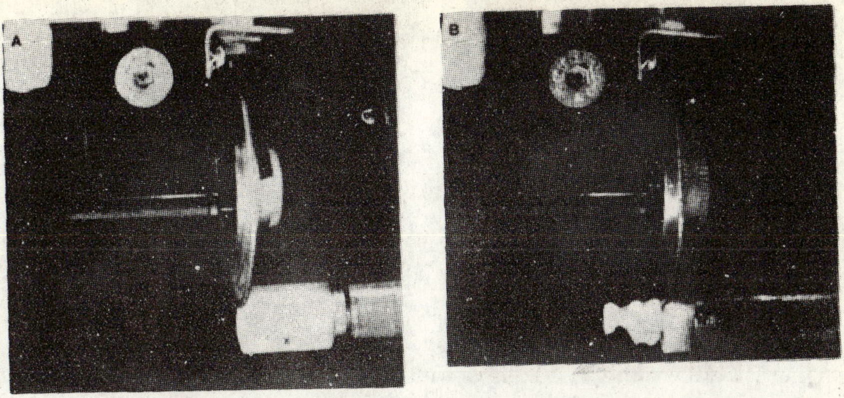

Fig (13) - Computer controls small milling device which cuts restoration out of block rotates as it moves forward into cutting wheel. Cutting wheel moves up and down as needed to form inlay.

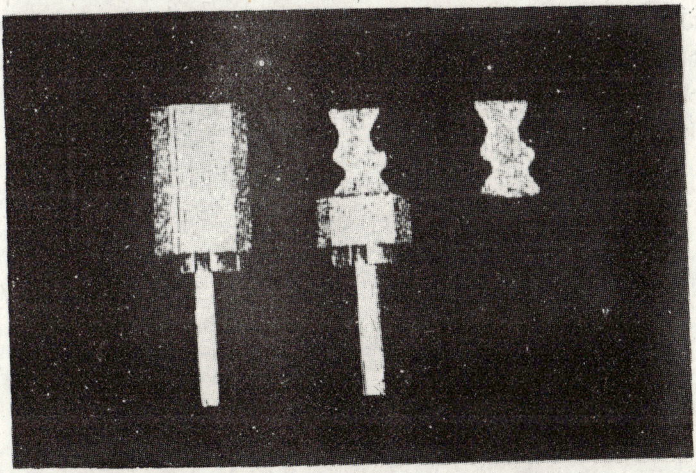

Fig (14) - CAD-CAM ceramicblock before milling (left) at an intermediate stage of milling (center), and after milling and removal, of the inlay from the mounting stub (right).

There are five basic stages in the fabrication : (1) Computerized surface digitization, (2) Computer aided design, (3)Computer aided manufacturing, (4) Computer aided esthetics, and (5) Computer aided finishing.

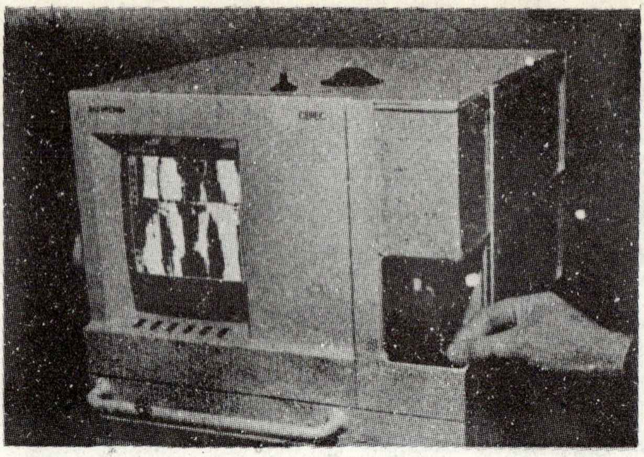

'ig (15) - **Milling operation usually takes** 5 to 7 minutes tocomplete. Inlay s then removed from milling chamber and is ready for try-in.

Earlier monolithic restorations (Uniform shade) were only ivailable from CAD/CAM technique, but now some latitude in :olour selection is possible; More over external shading or layering vith feldspathic porcelain may be done to achieve better esthetics.

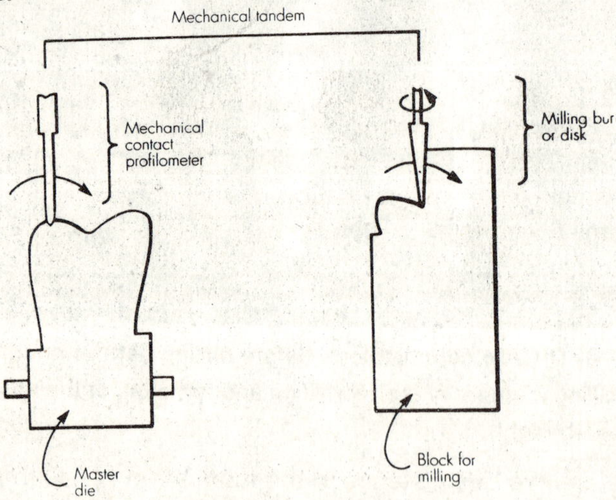

Fig (16) - Schematic representation of copy milling.

Pertinent information on copy milling is given in table 1.

LEUCITE REINFORCED CERAMICS :

Commercially it is available as Optec HSP: The material contains leucite developed by crystallization in situ by the manufacturer. Its dispersion strengthens the glass. This material does not require separate core and veneering ceramics.

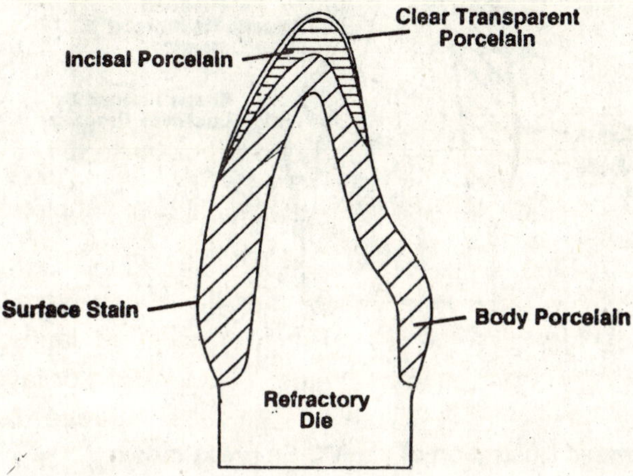

Fig (17) - Schematic illustration of an Optec HSP crown

Fabrication :

The conventional condensation and sintering is done on a special semi-permeable die at a temperature of 1020°C.

PRESSABLE CERAMICS :

The heat press technique was developed following innovative injection moulded shrink free ceramics in 1983 at University of Zurich. Both leucite reinforced feldspathic porcelains and leucite enriched glass - ceramics were made available for use with this technique.

IPS Empress : It is a pre-cerammed leucite enriched glass - ceramic. The pre-ceramming process saves time for the dentist / technician.

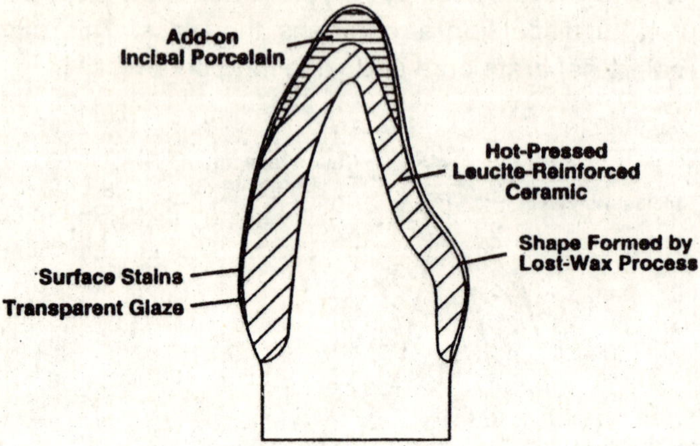

Fig (18) - Schematic illustration of asnIPS Empress crown.

The manufacturer supplies the pre-cerammed material as ingots to be heat moulded under pressure in a special mould with alumina plunger.

Heat-Press Injection Moulded technique :

Two individual dies of the working tooth are made for wax up and trial. The wax up and die are invested in the specially designed cylindrical mould. The pre-heated ingot (1150°c) is placed in the mould opening and the alumina plunger positioned over it. The entire assembly is placed in the pre-heated, fully adjustable automatic furnace and at a temperature of 1050°C (if no layering is required) or 1180°C (if layering is required) & 0.3 - 0.4 MPa pressure is applied (5 bar)for 30-40 mts. This can also be used for shad'ng or glazing procedures and will result in further improvement of strength due to crystal growth. If layering is to be done, 0.3 mm of the full contoured restoration is cutback and feldspathic porcelain can be layered.

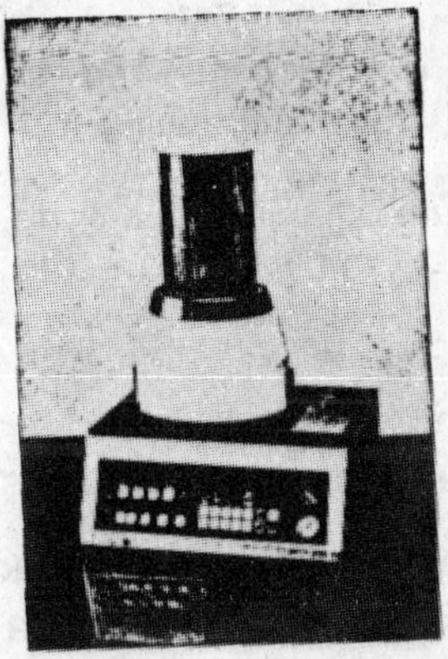

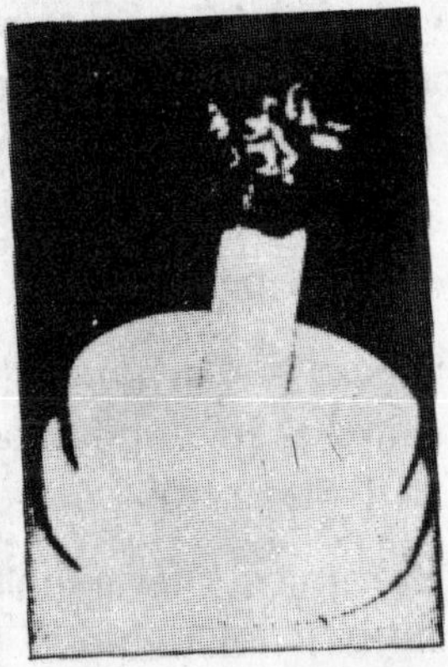

Fig (19) - (Left) The IPS-Empress EP 500 furnace is especially designed for this system. Displays show different characteristics of the press furnace

Fig (19-a) - (Right)The inlays must be waxed and placed on a specially designed cylindrical crucible former.

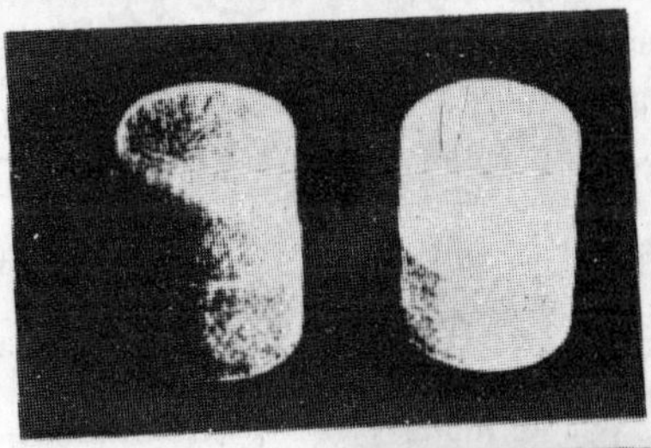

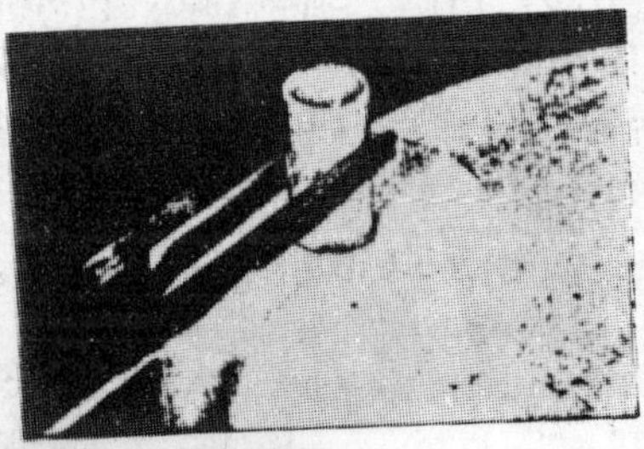

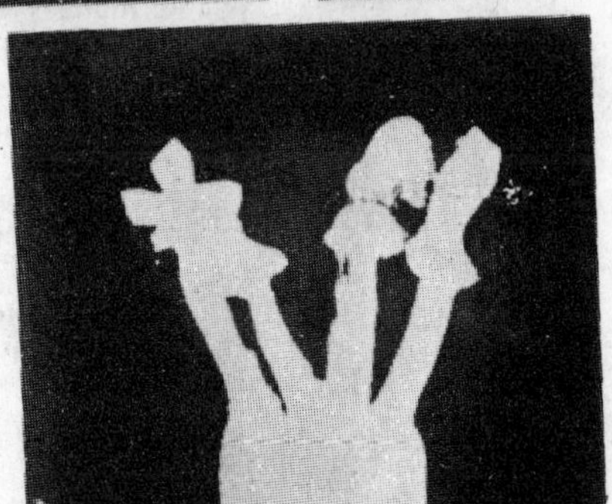

Fig (20) - Ceramic ingots are preshaded and precerammed. For the inlay technique, translucent material is used.

Fig (20-a) - After filling the cylindrical opening with an already preheated ceramic ingot and an Al2O3 pushing rod, the cast must be placed into the preheated Empress furance. The aluminium oxidepushing rod is used to transfer the pressure to the ceramic material.

Fig (20-b) - After the press procedure, the inlays are devested and prepared for further treatments.

Optec Pressable Ceramic : This is a modified feldspathic porcelain with increased leucite content. The particle size of leucite is decreased, but the content increased to improve the strength.

Pressable ceramics offer excellent fit owing to the fact that the volumetric shrinkage of ceramic is compensated by a matched expansion of the special mould.

INFILTRATED CERAMICS :

A strong ceramic oxide infused with glass yields infiltrated ceramics. The stronger ceramic is intentionally sintered with porosity which will later, by capillary action, be sealed with molten glass. Fine grain particles of ceramic oxide are mixed with water to form a suspension called slip.

Inceram : Either alumina or spinel is slip cast to be infiltrated with matching glass

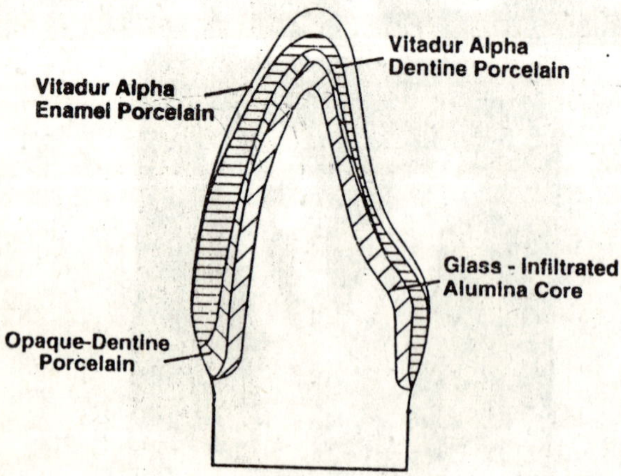

Fig (21) - Schematice illustration of an In-Ceram crown.

Slip Casting and Glass Infusion :

On a gypsum die the slip of ceramic oxide is baked at 1120°c for 10hrs. Glass powder is painted over the porous ceramic coping and baked at 1100°c for 4 hrs.

This is used as a strong core to be veneered by feldspathic porcelain.

In ceram spinel is more translucent and less stronger than Inceram alumina.

Traditional etching of Inceram is not possible. Hence a new method BERS (Batman's etch retentive system) has been introduced. In this plastic chips are incorporated on the fitting surface and burnt off to leave pits that are retentive. But this has been found to reduce the flexural strength of the material. Hence sand blasting and resin cementation is recommended.

NEW LOW FUSING CERAMICS :

Duceram LFC :

This is a hydrothermal low fusing ceramic composed of amorphous glass containing OH ions. This increases the density, flexural strength and fracture resistance and decreases the hardness. The strength increase is attributed to OH ion exchange that promotes crack healing.

Fabrication : 2 layers of Duceram are to be applied. The base layer is a leucite porcelain used for metal-ceramic purposes. This is applied on a refractory die. Condensation is done and sintering carried out at 930°C. The superficial duceram layer is of the LFC type, condensed and sintered at 660°C.

They are highly polishable in the oral cavity and hence do not require glazing. Other low fusing ceramics are the Golden gate system, Ducera gold, Fenesse and Procera All-ceram.

PHYSICAL AND MECHANICAL PROPERTIES AND OTHER CONSIDERATIONS FOR VARIOUS CERAMICS

MATERIAL	FLEXURAL STRENGTH (MPa)	COMPRESSIVE STRENGTH (MPa)	TENSILE STRENGTH (MPa)	HARDNESS (KHN)	LCTE (ppm/^{o}c)	MODULUS OF ELASTICITY	BIOCOMPATIBILITY	AESTHETICS	OTHERS
FELDSPATHIC PORCELAIN	68.9	344	34.4	460	6.0	12.0×10^5 psi	Excellent	Excellent	
ALUMINA	379	2180	138				Excellent	Opaque	
ALUMINOUS PORCELAINS VITADURN	125						Excellent	Opaque	
HI - CERAM	155						Excellent	Opaque	Special refractory die needed for fabrication.
SHRINK-FREE CERAMICS CERESTORE	120	1048			5.6	1.23×10^5 Mpa	Excellent	Good	The injection moulded technique provides excellent fit due to the volumetric increase caused by formation of aluminosilicate and spinel.
AL-CERAM	225				5.6	1.23×10^5 Mpa	Excellent	Good	
MAGNESIA CORE CERAMIC	131-269				13.0		Excellent	Opaque	Magnesium Silicate (forsterite) formation in-situ augments the strength.

MATERIAL	FLEXURAL STRENGTH (MPa)	COMPRESSIVE STRENGTH (MPa)	TENSILE STRENGTH (MPa)	HARDNESS (KHN)	LCTE (ppm/^{o}c)	MODULUS OF ELASTICITY	BIOCOMPATIBILITY	AESTHETICS	OTHERS
CASTABLE CERAMICS DICOR	152	620		362	7.2	10.2×10^5 psi	Excellent	Good	Transformation of transparent cast glass into crystalline glass-ceramic retains the translucency and enhances the strength. Excellent fit is another advantage as the lost wax technique is used.
CERA PEARL	70			Same as Tooth			Excellent	Excellent	The hydroxyapatite crystals arranged irregularly in the matrix making the final restoration more esthetic than other glass - ceramics. All glass ceramics are etchable and bondable to tooth.
MACHINABLE CERAMICS DICOR MGC	147			330	6.4	6.8×10^5 mPa	Excellent	Fair	
CERELC VITA BLOC MARK I	93			Similar to felds - pathic porcelain	Similar to felds - pathic porcelain	Similar to felds - pathic porcelain	Excellent	Good	Marginal gap of all machined restorations are more than laboratory made restorations. Exposure of the resin cement through this gap leads to wear and marginal ditching.

MATERIAL	FLEXURAL STRENGTH (MPa)	COMPRESSIVE STRENGTH (MPa)	TENSILE STRENGTH (MPa)	HARDNESS (KHN)	LCTE (ppm/^{o}c)	MODULUS OF ELASTICITY	BIOCOMPATIBILITY	AESTHETICS	OTHERS
CERELC VITA BLOC MARK II	152			Same as tooth			Excellent	Good	
CELAY - COPY MILLED RESTORATION	152			Same as tooth			Excellent	Good	Copy milling uses a replica of restoration in wax, stone, plastic or metal as a guide for a milling machine. The surface of the replica is traced by turning the pattern and touching it with similar form fingerguides. The positions of the pattern and finger guide are used to adjust the positions of the block of restorative material and the milling tool.
PRESSABLE CERAMICS IPS EMPRESS	126	750-814		More than feldspathic porcelain			Excellent	Excellent	Heat press technique provides excellent fitting and translucent restoration. Subsequent heat treatments increase the strength to 160-182 Mpa for IPs-Empress.
OPTEC PRESABLE CERAMIC (OPC)	165			More than feldspathic porcelain			Excellent	Excellent	

MATERIAL	FLEXURAL STRENGTH (MPa)	COMPRESSIVE STRENGTH (MPa)	TENSILE STRENGTH (MPa)	HARDNESS (KHN)	LCTE (ppm/°c)	MODULUS OF ELASTICITY	BIOCOMPATIBILITY	AESTHETICS	OTHERS
LEUCITE REIN FORCED CERAMICS	146			More than feldspathic porcelain			Excellent	Excellent	Core is not needed for this restoration
NEW LOW FUSING CERAMICS	110			Same as tooth			Excellent	good	Lowest fusing ceramic available
DULERAM LFC PROCERA	360						Excellent	Opaque	High purity alumina is dry pressed over enlarged machine duplicated die, removed and sintered at 1550°c for 1 hr.
MODIFIED PROCERA	375						Excellent	Opaque	Fabrication is done by contact digital scanning of gypsum die rather than machine duplication. Computer data is loaded. The procera software package manipulates the scanned image, defines finish lines, coping thickness, collar design etc. Data is transferred by modem to remote manufacturer.
INFILTRATED CERAMICS IN-CERAM ALUMINA	450	964		Same as feldspathic porcelain			Excellent	Opaque	Infiltrated ceramics are not etchable.
IN-CERAM SPINEL	340			Same as feldspathic porcelain			Excellent	Good	

REFERENCES :

1. Derek W. Jones, Ceramics, Dental Clinics of North America (DCNA) October, 1985, 29 (4) :
2. John W. Mc Lean, The Science and Art of Ceramics, Vol. I. Quintessence Publn., 1979.
3. Ralph W. Phillips, Skinner's Science of Dental Materials, 9th ed. 1992.
4. K.J. Anusavice, Phillip's Science of Dental materials, 10th ed. 1996.
5. Marc A. Rosenblum, Allan Schullman, A review of all-ceramic restorations, JADA, march, 1997, 128 (3); p-297.
6. G.J. Christensen, Why All-ceramic restorations?

   JADA, October, 1997, 128 (10); p-1453
7. Robert J. Cronin, David R. Cagna, An update on Fixed Prosthodontics, JADA, April, 1997, 128(4); p-432
8. Mak, Qualtrough, and Burke, The effect of different ceramic materials on the fracture resistance of dentin bonded crowns, Quint Int. 28(3); p-197.
9. Julie A. Hollaway, I.L. Denry, S.F. Rosenstiel, Surface layer chracterization after dual ion - exchange of a leucite reinforced porcelain, Int. Journal of Prostho., March / April 1997, Vol 10 (2)
10. Patrick J. Steiner, J.R. Kelly, A.A. Guiseppetti, Compatibility of Cermaic - Ceramic systems for fixed prosthodontics, Int- Journal of prostho; Jul/Aug. 1997, Vol 10 (4); p-375
11. M.H. Ramp, Shiro Suzuki, C.F. Cox, W.R. Lacefield, D.C. Koth, Evaluation of wear : Enamel opposing 3 ceramic materials and a gold alloy, J.P.D., May 1997,77 (5); p-523.
12. Peter yamen, S.R. Qazi, T.B. Dennison & M.E. Razzoog, Effect of adding opaque porcelain on the final colour of porcelain laminates, JPD, Feb.1997, 77(2), P -136.
13. Mauro Fradeani & Augusto Aquilano, Clinical experience with Empress crowns. Int-Journal of Prostho. May/June 1997, Vol.10-(3), P-241.

14. D.J. Wood, W.L. Buff, B. J. Millar & S.M. Dunne Preliminary investigation of a novel retentive system for hydrofluoric acid etch resistant, dental ceramics: JPD, September, 1997 78(3). P-275.

15. Christian Lehner, Stephan Studer, Urs Brodbeck and Peter Scharer, Short term results of IPS empress full porcelain crowsn. J.O.P., March 6(1), P-120

16. J. Fischer, C. Kuntze & F. Lampert, Modified partial coverage ceramics for interior teeth - A new restorative method, Quint Int., May 1997, 28(5). P-293.

17. Mormann WH & Bindl A, The new creativity in Ceramic restoratons ; Dental CAD/CIM Quint. Int 27, 821-8, 996 Dental Abstracts, July / Aug. 1997, Vol. 42 # 4, P. 174

18. Herber. T. Schillingberg, Richard Jacob, & Susan E. Brackett, Fundamentals of Tooth Preparations for cast metal & porcelain reotoration, quintessence publishing. 1991.

19. William F.P. Malone, & David. L. Koth, Tylman's theory & Practice of Fixed Prosthodontics, 8th ed. IEA Publication, 1989.

20. J.K. Dong, H. Lathy, A. Wohlwend & P. Scharer, Heat pressed Ceramics: Technology and Strength, The Int. J. of Prostho: Vol. 5 # 1; p - 9-15, 1992.

21. Lother Probster, Compressive strength of two modern All-Ceramic Crowns, Int. J. Prosthodont 1992, 5, # 5, P-409-414.